MCQs in Neurology and Neurosurgery for Medical Students

Edited by

IBRAHIM NATALWALA

MBBS, MSc (Distinction)
Core Surgery (Plastics)
Health Education West Midlands

and

AMMAR NATALWALA

MBChB, BSc (Hons), MRCS (Eng)
Department of Neurosurgery
Queen's Medical Centre, Nottingham

Foreword by

E GLUCKSMAN
FRCP, FRCSEd, FCEM
Consultant in Emergency Medicine

Radcliffe Publishing
London • New York

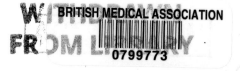

Radcliffe Publishing Ltd
St Mark's House
Shepherdess Walk
London N1 7LH
United Kingdom

www.radcliffehealth.com

British Library Cataloguing in Publication Data

A catalogue record for this book is available from the British Library.

ISBN-13: 978 184619 483 2

The paper used for the text pages of this book
is FSC® certified. FSC (The Forest Stewardship
Council®) is an international network to promote
responsible management of the world's forests.

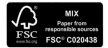

Typeset by Darkriver Design, Auckland, New Zealand
Printed and bound by Hobbs the Printers, Totton, Hants, UK

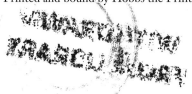

Contents

Contents

Foreword

This book provides you with MCQs covering important aspects of neuro-science to help you not only to learn the basics but also to appreciate how to apply your knowledge to clinical practice. The chapters are arranged so that a series of questions is followed by the answers with explanations, so the answers are easy to link to the questions. The authors use diagrams and images to good effect to complement the text.

This book can be used to highlight strengths in your knowledge, but just in case there are any weaknesses, the authors have referenced their answers to help you identify further reading.

One of the particularly interesting approaches taken by the authors has been to seek contributions from medical students and doctors in the early phases of their training. Their perspective has helped to influence the material included and adds clarity to the way information is presented and organised.

I hope you find this book informative and useful during undergraduate education through postgraduate training and beyond as a handy reference as part of life-long learning.

E Glucksman FRCP, FRCSEd, FCEM
Consultant in Emergency Medicine
September 2013

Preface

In examining disease, we gain wisdom about anatomy and physiology and biology. In examining the person with disease, we gain wisdom about life.

Oliver Sacks

As a medical student, neurology and neurosurgery can be extremely daunting specialties to learn about. Often as a student I used to wonder where to start. I realised that the greater the depth of neurology or neurosurgery I studied, the more fascinating yet overwhelming it became. The pragmatic approach to learning neurology and neurosurgery is to start with the basic knowledge and know it well, as it will be used in your everyday practice right the way from a junior doctor to a senior consultant.

This MCQ book has been designed to cover the most important basic elements of neuroanatomy, neurophysiology and neuroradiology through to stroke, central nervous system lesions and malignancies. The questions are followed by detailed answers that will help to create a better familiarity with each topic. There are also some essential diagrams, such as of visual field defects, since these topics tend to be college favourites. The answers are also referenced to high-quality publications so that it is possible to read around the topic further, and we highly recommend this!

Ideally, this book should be used as a learning tool before exams to test your depth of knowledge and revise the areas where it may be lacking. However, we have designed the book so questions are grouped into particular themes, primarily to allow easy and quick referencing when required. We hope these questions and detailed answers will enable you to achieve success in your exams and in your future clinical practice.

Ibrahim Natalwala
September 2013

About the editors

Ibrahim Natalwala

Ibrahim is a Core Surgical Trainee in the West Midlands with a plastic surgery themed training programme. He completed his clinical training from King's College London and also graduated with a Distinction in an intercalated MSc in Clinical Neurosciences. As a medical student, he completed a 3-week placement at Jikei University Tokyo in general surgery and neurosurgery.

He finished his Academic Foundation Training at the University Hospital of North Staffordshire where he spent a 4-month rotation in epidemiological research at the Arthritis Research UK Primary Care Centre at Keele University.

Ammar Natalwala

Mr Natalwala is currently a trainee in the Department of Neurosurgery at the Queen's Medical Centre in Nottingham. He graduated from Birmingham University in 2009 and completed an intercalated BSc degree in Neurosciences at King's College London in 2006. His Foundation Year training was in Southampton and this included a 4-month academic post in Neurosurgery. He then spent a year in Sheffield doing Neurosurgery before starting run-through training in Nottingham.

About the contributors

Surajit Basu

Mr Basu is a Consultant Neurosurgeon at the Queen's Medical Centre in Nottingham and leads the functional neurosurgery service. His sub-specialist interests include deep brain stimulation, epilepsy surgery, neurosurgery for chronic pain and awake tumour surgeries.

Indira Natarajan

Dr Natarajan is a consultant physician in stroke and general medicine at the University Hospital of North Staffordshire.

Sarmad Al-Araji

Dr Sarmad Al-Araji is currently a Foundation Year 1 doctor at the University Hospital of North Staffordshire. He achieved his MBChB from the Keele University School of Medicine. His interest in neurology was confirmed during his 8-week placement in neurology as a fourth-year medical student. His experience in neurology includes a special selected module in neurology at the end of the fourth year, a 4-week elective in neurology at Vancouver General Hospital and a 4-week elective in neuroradiology at Charing Cross Hospital. He also undertook a 4-month rotation in stroke, during which he presented a poster as part of the European Stroke Conference in London in May 2013. He will continue his neurological and neurosurgical training during Foundation Year 2.

James Turner

Dr James Turner is a Foundation Year 1 doctor currently working at the University Hospital of North Staffordshire. He took an interest in neurology in his fourth year of medical school at Keele University. He has completed a 3-month rotation in neurosurgery at the University Hospital of North Staffordshire.

Harriet Williamson

Dr Harriet Williamson gained an MBChB with honours from the Keele University School of Medicine (2007–12). She is currently undertaking her

Foundation training at the South Thames London Deanery. At present she works at the Queen Elizabeth Hospital Woolwich.

Joshua Kearsley

Joshua is a fourth-year medical student at the Keele University School of Medicine. He has also recently completed an intercalated BSc in medical sciences at Hull York Medical School (2012–13).

Mahdi Saleh

Mahdi is a fourth-year medical student at the Keele University School of Medicine. He is co-founder of the Keele Neurology Society and has twice been elected member of the executive committee of the Keele Surgical Society. He will undertake his elective at Johns Hopkins University in the Neurosurgical Unit.

Yashashwi Sinha

Yashashwi is a fourth-year medical student at the Keele University School of Medicine. He has been accepted to undertake an intercalated MRes in stem cells and tissue engineering at Newcastle University (2013–14). His interest in neurology stems from dissection classes and seeing neurological disorders in practice during his clinical years.

Daniel Weinberg

Daniel is a fourth-year medical student at the Keele University School of Medicine. Having been intrigued by neurology and neurosurgery in his early clinical years, he is also co-founder of the Keele Neurology Society. The Keele Neurology Society aims to provide extra teaching and to encourage new interest within the subject area. Neurology continues to interest him as a logical branch of medicine, which is something he seeks in any medical or surgical specialty.

Queen's Medical Centre, Nottingham

We would like to thank the Radiology and Ophthalmology Departments at Queen's Medical Centre in Nottingham for providing the computed tomography and magnetic resonance images for this publication.

Abbreviations

AChR-Ab	acetylcholine receptor antibodies
AED	anti-epileptic drug
AIDP	acute inflammatory demyelinating polyradiculopathy
ALS	amyotrophic lateral sclerosis
CNS	central nervous system
CPP	cerebral perfusion pressure
CRAO	central retinal artery occlusion
CSDH	chronic subdural haematoma
CSF	cerebrospinal fluid
CT	computed tomography
CTS	carpal tunnel syndrome
DIND	delayed ischaemic neurological deficit
DM1	myotonic dystrophy type 1
DNA	deoxyribonucleic acid
EEG	electroencephalography
FVC	forced vital capacity
GABA	gamma-aminobutyric acid
GBS	Guillain–Barré syndrome
GCS	Glasgow Coma Scale
GMB	glioblastoma multiforme
GPi	globus pallidus interna
HD	Huntington's disease
HIV	human immunodeficiency virus
ICP	intracranial pressure
LEMS	Lambert–Eaton myasthenic syndrome
LGS	Lennox–Gastaut syndrome
MAP	mean arterial pressure
MCQs	multiple-choice questions
MG	myasthenia gravis
MND	motor neurone disease
MRI	magnetic resonance imaging

MS	multiple sclerosis
NIV	non-invasive ventilation
NMDA	N-methyl-D-aspartate
NMS	neuroleptic malignant syndrome
PAN	polyarteritis nodosa
PLS	primary lateral sclerosis
PPRF	paramedian pontine reticular formation
RAPD	relative afferent pupillary defect
SAH	subarachnoid haemorrhage
SIADH	syndrome of inappropriate antidiuretic hormone secretion
SNc	substantia nigra pars compacta
SNr	substantia nigra pars reticularis
WBC	white blood cell
WHO	World Health Organization

Dedicated to our parents
Dr Siraj Natalwala and Mrs Shamim Natalwala

1

Autoimmune conditions

Q1 Angela is a 43-year-old receptionist who presents to her GP complaining of weakness in her legs that makes it difficult for her to stand up from a chair. On neurological examination, her reflexes are diminished. Angela has a medical history of small cell lung carcinoma. The GP suspects that a paraneoplastic syndrome is causing these symptoms. Creatine kinase is normal. What is the most likely diagnosis?

a. Hypercalcaemia
b. Hyperthyroidism
c. Mononeuritis multiplex
d. Polymyositis
e. Lambert–Eaton myasthenic syndrome (LEMS)

Q2 With regard to myasthenia gravis (MG), which of the following statements are true and which are false?

a. It is a heterogeneous immunological disease.
b. It is characterised clinically by the presence of ptosis, muscle weakness that improves with increased activity and worsens with rest and fatigue.
c. LEMS is caused by antibodies binding to voltage-gated calcium ion channels in the presynaptic membrane.
d. Plasma exchange and intravenous immunoglobulin G should be the first line of treatment in patients with MG.
e. It is essential to check the thymus in a patient presenting with MG.

Q3 A 45-year-old man presents to the A&E department complaining of pain and loss of vision in the left eye. He has no other neurological symptoms and no ongoing medical problems (e.g. hypertension, diabetes). On fundoscopy, the image shown here was seen.

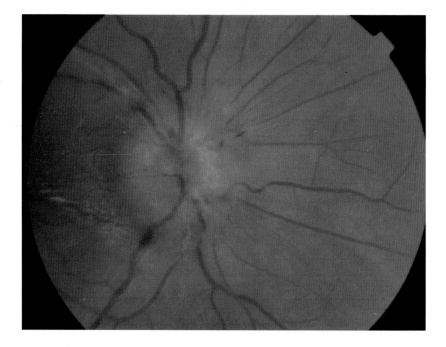

PART A

The appearance of the fundus shown is consistent with which of the following?

a. Normal appearance

b. Optic disc atrophy

c. Papilloedema

d. Hypertensive retinopathy

e. Macular degeneration

PART B

The clinical findings suggested optic neuritis; a diagnosis of multiple sclerosis (MS) was suspected and a magnetic resonance imaging (MRI) scan of the brain was subsequently performed. A white matter lesion was identified. What is the best treatment for this patient?

a. Azathioprine

b. Mitoxantrone

c. Intravenous immunoglobulin

d. Oral corticosteroid

e. None

After a successful recovery with the medication, several weeks later the patient returned to hospital, this time complaining of weakness in both legs. On clinical examination, it was found there was loss of sensation and he was incontinent. A repeat MRI scan showed another white matter lesion had developed. The clinical results demonstrated both dissemination in space and time as described by McDonald and colleagues;[1] hence the diagnosis of MS was confirmed.

PART C

With regard to the course of MS, which of the following statements are true and which are false?

a. Only 15% of people are first diagnosed with relapsing remitting MS.

b. If a patient shows deterioration for a period of at least 3 months, they have moved onto secondary progressive MS.

c. Approximately 85% of those diagnosed with relapsing remitting MS will go on to develop secondary progressive MS after 15 years of being diagnosed.

d. Men are as equally at risk of developing primary progressive MS as women.

Q4 Which of the following statements regarding autoimmune inflammatory myopathies such as polymyositis and dermatomyositis are true and
which are false?

 a. Muscle weakness is characteristically distal and symmetrical with
 most people having an element of myalgia.

 b. Muscle biopsies containing cytotoxic T-cells encircling non-
 necrotic myofibres are pathognomic for polymyositis.

 c. A heliotrope rash is specifically related to inclusion body myositis.

 d. Autoimmune myopathies are associated with increased risk of
 cancer.

 e. Dermatomyositis responds well to steroid therapy.

Q5 Which of the following most accurately describes the Uhthoff phenomenon in MS?

 a. Presence of an electric shock–like sensation down the spine upon
 flexion of the neck

 b. Worsening of symptoms during times when body temperature
 rises

 c. Persistent involuntary flickering of small bundles of the facial
 musculature

 d. Intense, unpredictable unilateral facial pain that is sharp in
 character

Q6 A 24-year-old man visits his GP because of increasing muscle weakness
in his lower extremities – this weakness started a couple of days ago. His
vital signs include a blood pressure of 94/62 mmHg, respiratory rate of
27 breaths per minute and a temperature of 36.9°C. Medical history
includes a severe gastroenteritis that he recently recovered from. The
GP suspects an acute inflammatory demyelinating polyradiculopathy
and arranges for a lumbar puncture. What cerebrospinal fluid (CSF)
findings are characteristic of this syndrome?

 a. Increased protein with a near-normal cell count

 b. Increased protein with an increased cell count

 c. Normal protein with a normal cell count

 d. Normal protein levels with an increased cell count

 e. Normal protein levels with a decreased cell count

Answers

A¹

Correct answer is E – LEMS

Small cell lung carcinoma can produce a range of paraneoplastic syndromes, of which LEMS would be the most likely in this case. This is due to the proximal muscle weakness that Angela is experiencing.[2] LEMS is an autoimmune disorder in which antibodies are directed against the presynaptic voltage-gated calcium channels. This results in a failure to release enough acetylcholine at the neuromuscular junction. In MG, it is the postsynaptic acetylcholine receptors that are affected. Therefore, clinically patients with LEMS and MG both experience muscle weakness. The difference, is that in LEMS sustained muscle effort leads to improvement in weakness whereas in MG prolonged effort is very difficult as fatigue progressively worsens. Trunk and legs are most often affected in LEMS, autonomic dysfunction can occur and hyporeflexia is typical on neurological examination.[3] Polymyositis is an inflammatory condition which predominantly causes pain and weakness in the proximal muscles. Patients will have a raised creatine kinase. Diagnosis is usually confirmed using electromyography and muscle biopsy. Mononeuritis multiplex would present with a painful, asymmetrical, asynchronous sensory and motor peripheral neuropathy involving isolated damage to at least two separate nerve areas.[4]

A²

a. TRUE – MG is essentially an autoimmune disorder, of which there can be paraneoplastic and non-paraneoplastic forms, and in which patients can be positive for either acetylcholine receptor antibodies (AChR-Ab) or muscle-specific receptor tyrosine kinase antibodies (MuSK-Ab).[5]
b. FALSE – The weakness worsens with activity since there is such a limited amount of acetylcholine receptors available. Other symptoms may include a change in the patient's voice, diplopia (note that ocular

signs are not common in LEMS), dull facial expression (almost as if there is paralysis), and if there is bulbar involvement then eating, drinking and breathing may also be affected.

c. TRUE – The inability of the voltage-gated calcium ion channels to open means that insufficient quantities of acetylcholine are released into the synaptic cleft and therefore the postsynaptic membrane may not depolarise, thus causing muscle weakness. LEMS is particularly associated with small cell carcinoma of the lung.[6]

d. FALSE – It should be anticholinesterase drugs such as neostigmine or pyridostigmine. Plasma exchange is recommended in severe cases and both intravenous immunoglobulin and plasma exchange can be used in exacerbations.[7]

e. TRUE – Patients may have a thymoma (causing the symptoms) that may be necessary to remove surgically, although there is no guarantee that this will lead to remission of the MG.[8]

A3

PART A
Correct answer is C – Papilloedema

Fundoscopy shows optic disc swelling consistent with papilloedema. In optic disc atrophy, the optic disc would appear shrunken and paler. Hypertensive retinopathy is due to chronic excessive hypertension, and changes to the retina include arteriolar narrowing, arteriovenous crossings, cotton wool spots, vessel sclerosis and haemorrhage.

PART B
Correct answer is D – Oral corticosteroid

According to the National Institute for Health and Care Excellence guidelines, oral or intravenous corticosteroid therapy is indicated in the treatment of optic neuritis. Steroids help to reduce inflammation and thus increase recovery, although it is recommended to limit corticosteroid treatment to more severe symptoms (where the relapse is painful or disabling) in order to avoid the side effects of steroid therapy. The other drugs are disease-modifying agents and are only indicated in MS patients with relapsing episodes and after full discussion and consideration of all the risks.[9]

PART C

a. FALSE – Most people (approximately 85%) are initially diagnosed with relapsing remitting MS. This means a patient will experience an exacerbation of symptoms for a period of 24 hours or more followed by a period of remission where the inflammation subsides and symptoms recover; in the early stages, recovery is usually complete, although with repeated relapses recovery may only be partial.

b. FALSE – A minimum period of 6 months of deterioration must be evident.

c. FALSE – Approximately 50% of people with relapsing remitting disease will develop secondary progressive MS after 10 years, and this percentage increases to 65% after 15 years of diagnosis.

d. TRUE – Primary progressive MS is rarer and usually diagnosed in older patients. Patients tend to continually deteriorate from the time of diagnosis and may suffer attacks during the course of the disease.[10]

A4

a. FALSE – Muscle weakness is usually proximal and symmetrical and thus patients with autoimmune myopathies have difficulty getting up from chairs, climbing stairs or brushing their hair. Patients can have significant myalgia as a result of the inflammation. Creatine kinase is usually raised. Diagnosis is made using electromyography and muscle biopsy.

b. TRUE – Cytotoxic T-cells are characteristically found in muscle biopsies of those with polymyositis and lead to inflammation. Biopsies of muscle from patients with dermatomyositis typically show perifascicular atrophy as a result of perivascular antibody responses. In inclusion body myositis, there is amyloid deposition and this is seen on the biopsy as inclusion bodies.

c. FALSE – A heliotrope rash is a purplish discolouration around the eyes and is specific to dermatomyositis. Gottron's papules are also found in dermatomyositis and are erythematous changes on the dorsum of the hand over the metacarpophalangeal, proximal interphalangeal and distal interphalangeal joints.

d. TRUE – Dermatomyositis is particularly associated with ovarian, lung, pancreatic, stomach and colonic cancers. Polymyositis is most commonly associated with non-Hodgkin's lymphoma and lung and bladder cancers.

Have a look at the images in Garcia-Cruz and Garcia-Doval's article:[11]
www.nejm.org/doi/full/10.1056/NEJMicm1002816

e. TRUE – Although dermatomyositis and polymyositis usually respond well to steroid therapy, inclusion body myositis does not. Azathioprine, methotrexate or cyclophosphamide may be trialled in those patients not responding to steroid therapy.[12]

A5

a. FALSE – This is known as Lhermitte's sign. Although commonly associated with MS, it can also be seen in patients with compression of the spinal cord, vitamin B_{12} deficiency, trauma, Behçet's disease and transverse myelitis.

b. TRUE – Wilhelm Uhthoff first described it in the late nineteenth century. In demyelinated peripheral nerves, even a slight increase in temperature can lead to slowing or blocking of electrical impulses and this can make symptoms of MS significantly worse.

c. FALSE – This is known as facial myokymia.

d. FALSE – This is known as trigeminal neuralgia.

All of these answers are terms for ancillary symptoms in MS.[13]

A6

Correct answer is A – Increased protein with a near-normal cell count

Increased protein levels with a near-normal cell count in the CSF together with the history are highly suggestive of Guillain–Barré syndrome (GBS). This classic finding is also known as albuminocytologic dissociation. The syndrome is associated with recent infections that result in autoimmune attack of peripheral myelin due to molecular mimicry. *Campylobacter jejuni*, which causes a severe gastroenteritis, is a common antecedent to this syndrome. Inflammation and demyelination of ventral roots causes symmetric ascending muscle weakness beginning in the distal lower extremities. Paralysis of muscles required for respiration can occur if left untreated, leading to respiratory depression or even death. Autonomic dysfunction can result in cardiac arrhythmias as well as hypertension or hypotension.[14]

References

1. McDonald WI, Compston A, Edan G, *et al*. Recommended diagnostic criteria for multiple sclerosis: guidelines from the International Panel on the Diagnosis of Multiple Sclerosis. *Ann Neurol*. 2001; **50**(1): 121–7.

2. Mareska M, Gutmann L. Lambert–Eaton myasthenic syndrome. *Semin Neurol*. 2004; **24**(2): 149–53.

3. Vincent A. Autoimmune disorders of the neuromuscular junction. *Neurol India*. 2008; **56**(3): 305–13.

4. Longmore M, Wilkinson IB, Davidson EH, *et al*. *Oxford Handbook of Clinical Medicine*. 8th ed. New York, NY: Oxford University Press; 2010.

5. Carr AS, Cardwell CR, McCarron PO, *et al*. A systematic review of population based epidemiological studies in myasthenia gravis. *BMC Neurol*. 2010; **10**: 46.

6. Takamori M. Lambert–Eaton myasthenic syndrome: search for alternative autoimmune targets and possible compensatory mechanisms based on presynaptic calcium homeostasis. *J Neuroimmunol*. 2008; **201–2**: 145–52.

7. Skeie GO, Apostolski S, Evoli A, *et al*. Guidelines for treatment of autoimmune neuromuscular transmission disorders. *Eur J Neurol*. 2010; **17**(7): 893–902.

8. Kumar V, Kaminski HJ. Treatment of myasthenia gravis. *Curr Neurol Neurosci Rep*. 2011; **11**(1): 89–96.

9. National Institute for Health and Care Excellence. Multiple Sclerosis: management of multiple sclerosis in primary and secondary care; clinical guideline 8. London: NICE; 2003. www.nice.org.uk/nicemedia/pdf/cg008guidance.pdf (accessed 11 October 2012).

10. Multiple Sclerosis Society. *What is MS?* London: Multiple Sclerosis Society; 2012. Available at: www.mssociety.org.uk/what-is-ms (accessed 11 October 2012).

11. X. Garcia-Cruz A, Garcia-Doval I. Gottron's Papules and Dermatomyositis. *N Engl J Med*. 2010; **363**: e17.

12. Mammen AL. Autoimmune myopathies: autoantibodies, phenotypes and pathogenesis. *Nat Rev Neurol*. 2011; **7**(6): 343–54.

13. Fauci A, Braunwald E, Kasper D, *et al.*, editors. *Harrison's Principles of Internal Medicine*. 17th ed. New York, NY: McGraw-Hill; 2008. pp. 1261–2.

14. Frosch MP, Anthony DC, De Girolami U. The central nervous system. In: Kumar V, Abbas AK, Fausto N, *et al. Robbins and Cotran Pathologic Basis of Disease, Professional Edition*. 8th ed. Philadelphia, PA: Saunders Elsevier; 2010.

2

Central nervous system lesions

Q1 Regarding syringomyelia, which of the following are true and which are false?

   a. It is caused by dissection of the ependyma of the central canal
   b. It typically presents in older persons
   c. Pain and temperature sensations are lost in the proximal arms
   d. It can present as a lower motor neurone lesion
   e. A patient can present with ptosis, pupillary constriction and problems with facial sweating

Q2 Internuclear opthalmoplegia is caused by damage or dysfunction of which part of the central nervous system (CNS)?

   a. Lateral geniculate nucleus
   b. Mammillary bodies
   c. Medial longitudinal fasciculus
   d. Dorsal columns
   e. Tegmentum

Q3 A 32-year-old man with Addison's disease is brought to the A&E department and is found to have life-threatening hyponatraemia. The hyponatraemia is immediately corrected. However, he finds it difficult to speak afterwards. The attending doctor confirms that the patient has diplopia and paralysis of his left leg in addition to his dysarthria. The patient soon loses consciousness. What is the most likely diagnosis that has occurred because of the rapid correction of the patient's hyponatraemia?

a. Central pontine myelinolysis

b. Wernicke–Korsakoff syndrome

c. Haemorrhagic infarct

d. Ischaemic infarct

e. Subarachnoid haemorrhage (SAH)

Q4 A 53-year-old lady is found having collapsed at home. On admission to hospital, she has a Glasgow Coma Scale score of 12 (Eye – 3, Speech – 4, Motor – 5). A post-contrast computed tomography (CT) scan of her head is performed, which demonstrates high attenuation in the sylvian fissures and the supra-sellar cistern. A CT angiogram demonstrates a large posterior communicating artery aneurysm.

Which of the following are common potential complications of her presenting condition?

a. Re-bleed, hydrocephalus, vasospasm, hypernatraemia

b. Re-bleed, hydrocephalus, vasospasm, hyponatraemia

c. Re-bleed, hydrocephalus, vasodilation, seizures

d. Re-bleed, hydrocephalus, vasodilation, hyponatraemia

Q5 Which of the following are signs of raised intracranial pressure (ICP)?

a. Optic disc atrophy

b. Trochlear (cranial nerve IV) palsies

c. Raised systolic blood pressure, narrow pulse pressure and tachycardia

d. Cheyne–Stokes respiration

e. Headaches which are made worse by coughing and straining

Q6 With regard to hydrocephalus, which of the following are true and which are false?

a. It can present in infancy as a result of an Arnold–Chiari malformation

b. The pathophysiology of hydrocephalus is entirely due to the over-production of CSF

c. CSF is produced in the ependymal cells of the choroid plexus

d. The process of returning CSF to the bloodstream is called pinocytosis

e. Normal pressure hydrocephalus usually presents in patients in their 60s as incontinence, aphasia and dementia

Answers

A¹

a. TRUE – Excess CSF in the central canal can lead to dissection of the ependyma (the epithelial-like layer lining the ventricles) and lead to a fluid-filled neuroglial cavity called a syrinx.

b. FALSE – It mainly presents in young adults and can be either congenital or acquired. In congenital syringomyelia there is usually an Arnold–Chiari malformation resulting from protrusion of the cerebellum below the foramen magnum (cerebellar tonsillar descent). Subsequently, this can lead to obstruction of CSF flow and formation of a syrinx. It can be acquired in several ways including trauma, meningitis and neoplasms.

c. TRUE – Pain and temperature sensation is lost in a shawl-like pattern. Pain and temperature sensation is carried in the spinothalamic tract. Typically, the dorsal columns are spared and thus the patient retains vibration, proprioception, touch and pressure sense.

d. TRUE – When the syrinx extends it can damage the lower motor neurones of the anterior horn cells, leading to wasting and weakness of the muscles of the hands (and may cause claw hand).

e. TRUE – Syringomyelia can cause Horner's syndrome due to damage to the sympathetic neurones in the intermediolateral cell column.[1]

A²

a. FALSE – Primary visual processing centre in the thalamus where information from the retinal ganglion cells is processed and its output is via the optic radiation.

b. FALSE – These are described as being part of the hypothalamus and the limbic system and thus are implicated in the function of memory. Pathology of the mammillary bodies is associated with amnesic syndromes. Also, damage as a result of Wernicke–Korsakoff syndrome may lead to anterograde memory loss.

c. TRUE – Internuclear opthalmoplegia is a clinical sign of extraocular muscle weakness related to the dysfunction of the medial longitudinal fasciculus tract. The medial longitudinal fasciculus pathways connect the paramedian pontine reticular formation (PPRF) and the abducens nucleus complex to the oculomotor nucleus, which allows conjugate eye movements to take place. The following image shows internuclear opthalmoplegia on clinical examination.

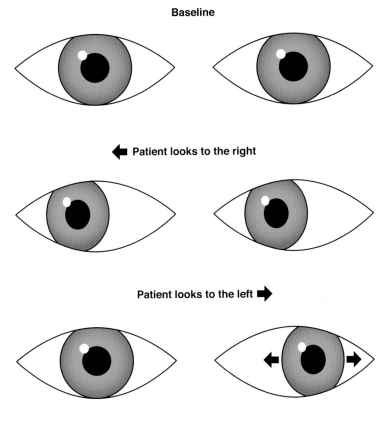

Baseline

◀ Patient looks to the right

Patient looks to the left ▶

Note: Left eye nystagmus,
         minimal right eye adduction

d. FALSE – They transmit sensory information including discriminative touch, pressure, vibration and proprioception via ascending pathways to the cortex.

e. FALSE – It is a general area within the brainstem; the tegmentum makes up the floor of the midbrain and the tectum makes up the ceiling. Multiple tracts run within these areas.

A³

Correct answer is A – Central pontine myelinolysis

Central pontine myelinolysis is a fatal complication that is due to rapid correction of hyponatraemia. An acute onset of paralysis, dysarthria, dysphagia, diplopia and eventual loss of consciousness may occur following correction. An MRI scan could show an abnormally increased signal in the pons due to myelinolysis. This condition occurs because of a rapid increase in serum tonicity in patients with severe hyponatraemia who have made intracellular compensations.[2] Expert advice should be sought when correcting hyponatraemia as different scenarios require different treatment patterns, for example, in rapid onset symptomatic hyponatraemia hypertonic saline may be considered but in asymptomatic hypovolaemic hyponatraemia 0.9% normal saline is used to raise serum sodium concentration by between 8 and 12 mmol/L in the first 24 hours.[3]

Wernicke–Korsakoff syndrome (answer B) is not related to rapid correction of hyponatraemia. It occurs as a result of vitamin B_1 deficiency.

A haemorrhagic infarct (answer C) does not occur due to rapid correction of hyponatraemia.

An ischaemic infarct (answer D) does not occur because of rapid correction of hyponatraemia.

A SAH (answer E) occurs most commonly as a result of a ruptured berry aneurysm in patients with *no history of trauma* (note that trauma to the head is the commonest cause of SAHs overall).

A⁴

Correct answer is B – Re-bleed, hydrocephalus, vasospasm, hyponatraemia

This patient has had an aneurysmal SAH. The common complications are re-bleed, hydrocephalus, vasospasm, hyponatraemia and seizures. Hypernatraemia and vasodilation are not complications of SAH.

The risk of re-bleed is 20%–30% in the first month after a SAH and stabilises to approximately 3% per year. Risk of re-bleed may be as high as 15% in the first 24 hours following a SAH. Prevention of re-bleed is performed via surgical clipping or endovascular coil embolisation of the aneurysm.

Clinical vasospasm can present with a reduced Glasgow Coma Scale score or delayed ischaemic neurological deficit (stroke) and is considered to occur as a result of irritation of the blood vessels by the subarachnoid blood. Radiological vasospasm is visible on angiography in 30%–70% of patients. Nimodipine, a calcium channel blocker, is used to prevent vasospasm and has been demonstrated to improve outcome in these patients. Triple H therapy (hypertension, hypervolaemia and haemodilution) is used to treat vasospasm and predominantly involves the administration of intravenous fluids and invasive blood pressure monitoring. More invasive methods – such as cerebral angioplasty or intra-arterial vasodilator therapy – can also be used to treat vasospasm in refractory cases. The aim of triple H therapy is to increase the mean arterial pressure (MAP) and thus cerebral perfusion pressure (CPP). This can be explained by the following formula which links MAP to CPP:

$$CPP = MAP - ICP$$

Acute hydrocephalus occurs in 20%–30% of SAH patients and may be treated with an external ventricular drain in the acute setting. In 18%–26% of surviving patients requiring permanent CSF diversion for chronic ventriculomegaly, a shunt can be inserted to divert the flow of CSF (e.g. ventriculoperitoneal shunt).[4]

The frequency of seizures following SAH has been reported to be between 6% and 18%. Routine use of anticonvulsants following SAH has not been proven useful. Hyponatraemia has a reported incidence of 10%–30% following SAH. It is important to determine the cause of this. It may be a result of syndrome of inappropriate antidiuretic hormone secretion (SIADH), cerebral salt wasting, or it may be caused by other systemic disease or iatrogenic fluid administration. The differential is important because the treatment for each is different. SIADH is treated by fluid restriction whereas cerebral salt wasting is treated with hydration, sodium replacement and sometimes fludrocortisone.[4,5]

A[5]

a. TRUE – Papilloedema occurs initially as a result of raised ICP leading to optic nerve oedema and eventually results in optic nerve atrophy if untreated.

b. FALSE – Abducens (cranial nerve VI) palsies are usually associated with raised ICP.

   c. FALSE – Cushing's reflex of raised systolic blood pressure, widened pulse pressure and bradycardia can be seen with raised ICP.

   d. TRUE – Damage to the cerebral hemispheres can lead to phases of rapid breathing followed by the absence of breathing.

   e. TRUE

Very important learning points:

$$K_{ICP} \sim V_{CSF} + V_{Bl} + V_{Br}$$

K_{ICP}	Constancy of ICP
V_{CSF}	Volume of CSF
V_{Bl}	Volume of blood
V_{Br}	Volume of brain

The constancy of intracranial pressure (K_{ICP}) is relative to the CSF, blood and brain volumes. The ICP is maintained by auto-regulation and one such mechanism involves monitoring the levels of CO_2. If these levels rise, then there is an increase in cerebral blood flow. This means in cases of severe head injury (where V_{bl} may be increased), if pCO_2 levels rise, vasodilatation of the cerebral arteries will cause increased cerebral blood flow and this will further increase V_{bl} and hence increase ICP. This will result in reduced cerebral perfusion pressures (thereby increasing the risk of ischaemia and stroke):

$$CPP = MAP - ICP$$

In order to keep CPPs between the required 60–160 mmHg pressure (the physiological limits where autoregulation is effective), patients are often hyperventilated to reduce $PaCO_2$ levels (aiming for a $PaCO_2$ of 4.0 to 4.5).

    In the case of a mass (such as a haematoma) compressing the brain and causing raised ICP, initially venous blood and CSF are displaced out of the cranial cavity. This allows the ICP to be maintained up to a point where the mass is approximately 100 mL in volume. If the mass enlarges further, it exceeds the critical level and the ICP then increases very rapidly as auto-regulation fails. In these patients, mannitol (a diuretic) can be used to reduce the ICP prior to more definitive neurosurgical intervention.[6]

A⁶

a. TRUE – An Arnold–Chiari malformation results in the cerebellar tonsils descending into the cervical canal. It is associated with spina bifida and can lead to syringomyelia. Other causes of infantile hydrocephalus include stenosis of the aqueduct of Sylvius and Dandy–Walker syndrome (cerebellar hypoplasia and obstruction to the outflow from the fourth ventricle).[7]

b. FALSE – Hydrocephalus results from an imbalance in production and reabsorption but also blockage of the CSF along its path.[8]

c. TRUE – CSF is produced in the cerebral ventricles containing the choroid plexus.[8]

d. TRUE – Arachnoid villi located in the superior sagittal sinus return CSF to the bloodstream within vacuoles. This process is called pinocytosis.[9]

e. FALSE – Normal pressure hydrocephalus in a patient usually causes incontinence, ataxia and dementia (Hakim's triad). A way to remember this is 'weird, wet and wobbly'. This is due to expansion of the ventricles distorting the fibres of the corona radiata.[7]

References

1. Snell RS. *Clinical Neuroanatomy*. 7th ed. Philadelphia, PA: Lippincott Williams & Wilkins; 2009.
2. Lampl C, Yazdi K. Central pontine myelinolysis. *Eur Neurol*. 2002; **47**(1): 3–10.
3. Sterns RH, Nigwekar SU, Hix JK. The treatment of hyponatremia. *Semin Nephrol*. 2009; **29**(3): 282–99.
4. Bederson JB, Connolly ES Jr, Batjer HH, *et al*. Guidelines for the management of aneurysmal subarachnoid hemorrhage: a statement for healthcare professionals from a special writing group of the Stroke Council, American Heart Association. *Stroke*. 2009; **40**(3): 994–1025.
5. Harrigan MR. Cerebral salt wasting syndrome: a review. *Neurosurgery*. 1996; **38**(1): 152–60.
6. Goldberg A, Stansby G. *Surgical Talk: revision in surgery*. 2nd ed. London: Imperial College Press; 2005.
7. Kumar P, Clark ML, editors. *Kumar & Clark's Clinical Medicine*. 7th ed. Edinburgh: Saunders Elsevier; 2009.
8. Fitzgerald MJT, Gruener G, Mtui E. *Clinical Neuroanatomy and Neuroscience*. 5th ed. Edinburgh: Elsevier Saunders; 2007.
9. Martin EA. *Concise Medical Dictionary*. 7th ed. Oxford: Oxford University Press; 2007.

3

Central nervous system neoplasms

Q1 Regarding CNS tumours, which of the following are true and which are false?

    a. The most common intracranial tumour is a glioma

    b. Primary CNS tumours in adults are most commonly found below the tentorium cerebelli

    c. A 'negative' CT scan of the head excludes intracranial tumours

    d. On first diagnosis, primary brain tumours are usually low grade

    e. Headaches and epilepsy are the most common presenting symptoms of a primary brain tumour

Q2 Which of the following cancers is responsible for the majority of brain metastases?

    a. Prostate cancer

    b. Lung cancer

    c. Pancreatic cancer

    d. Colorectal cancer

    e. Breast cancer

Q3 Regarding CNS tumours, which of the following are true and which are false?

a. Glioblastoma multiforme (GBM) is the most aggressive type of astrocytoma.

b. Pilocytic astrocytomas often affect older people but are curable by resection

c. Ependymomas can be found adjacent to the ventricles in many patients

d. Meningiomas are usually arachnoid mater based

e. CNS lymphomas are usually high-grade Hodgkin's lymphomas

Q4 A 79-year-old man is brought to the A&E department because of a prolonged seizure. An MRI scan of his head shows a mass in the right cerebral hemisphere and a biopsy shows pleomorphic tumour cells bordering a central area of necrosis. The tumour cells stain positive for glial fibrillary acid protein. The patient undergoes a tumour debulking procedure where carmustine wafers are inserted into the tumour cavity. What is the mechanism of action of the class of drugs that includes carmustine?

a. An alkylating agent that cross-links DNA

b. An antibiotic that intercalates DNA

c. An anti-metabolite that decreases DNA synthesis

d. A vinca alkaloid that inhibits microtubule formation

e. A monoclonal antibody directed against a specific tumour cell receptor

Q5 From the list of answers provided, select the most likely diagnosis that corresponds to its characteristic findings.

    i. GBM

   ii. Meningioma

  iii. Schwannoma

  iv. Oligodendroglioma

   v. Pilocytic astrocytoma

  vi. Medulloblastoma

 vii. Ependymoma

viii. Craniopharyngioma

  ix. Haemangioblastoma

   x. Metastatic tumour

a. A relatively rare tumour that is most often found in the frontal lobes. Characterised by a 'fried egg' appearance on histology consisting of round nuclei with a clear cytoplasm.

b. Multiple, well-circumscribed tumours commonly found at the grey–white matter junction.

c. The most common primary brain tumour with the worst prognosis. A characteristic 'pseudo-palisading' arrangement of tumour cells that surround a central area of necrosis.

d. A tumour that is usually localised to the vestibulocochlear nerve (cranial nerve VIII) and at the cerebellopontine angle – stains S-100 positive.

e. A tumour originating from parts of Rathke's pouch that can calcify and cause bitemporal hemianopia.

Answers

A¹

a. FALSE – Metastases account for over 50% of all adult brain tumours, and 10%–50% of patients with systemic malignancy develop brain metastases.[1] *Primary* malignant brain tumours constitute approximately 2% of all adult cancers and are therefore rare.[2] A glioma is a brain tumour that arises from glial cells and is therefore an umbrella term that incorporates astrocytomas, ependymomas and oligodendrogliomas. Apart from metastases and gliomas, other types of brain tumours include meningiomas, pituitary adenomas and nerve sheath tumours.

b. FALSE – The majority of primary CNS tumours are supratentorial in adults, while infratentorial tumours are more common in children.[2]

c. FALSE – CT scans, particularly without contrast, were found to have a false-negative rate of up to 10% in an audit of 324 patients with gliomas.[3] MRI with gadolinium contrast enhancement is the investigation of choice for intracranial neoplasm.[4]

d. FALSE – Glioblastomas are the most common primary brain tumours in adults, which are World Health Organization (WHO) grade IV, the highest grade.[5]

e. TRUE – Headaches and epilepsy are the most common first presenting symptoms; however, they are rarely found in isolation without other symptoms or signs.[3] Headaches are the most common symptom in malignant tumours, whereas for lower-grade gliomas the most common symptom is seizures. Other symptoms include memory loss/confusion, personality problems and focal neurological symptoms.

A²

Correct answer is B – Lung cancer

Lung cancer is responsible for the majority of brain metastases, with the remainder accounted for by breast, renal, colorectal and melanoma. Most commonly, brain metastases are found in patients already known to have cancer; however, they may be found at the same time or before the primary cancer is found.[6,7]

A³

a. TRUE – GBM is a WHO-classified grade IV tumour. They are ring-enhancing lesions and the tumour cells show marked pleomorphism, mitosis, necrosis and florid proliferation. There are four key properties of CNS tumours that must be considered when identifying the grade:
   1. their ability to exhibit mass effect in the cranium, thereby causing severe symptoms or even death
   2. their ability to infiltrate the surrounding tissues, hence making excision impossible
   3. the difficulty of surgical resection due to risk of loss of essential brain functions
   4. the ability of slow-growing tumours to progress to more aggressive forms.

Therefore, CNS tumours can be classed as high grade or low grade; high grade being rapidly growing and infiltrating (WHO grades III and IV), and low grade being slowly growing and potentially curable (WHO grades I and II). The main reason for identifying the grade of a CNS lesion is to predict its prognostic factor and consequently grade I tumours have the best prognosis and grade IV tumours have the worst.[8] The following table shows some common CNS tumours and their WHO grading. This table is adapted from Louis et al.[9] – please see the full article for a detailed version and further explanations.

Type of CNS tumour	WHO grading			
	I	II	III	IV
Pilocytic astrocytoma	●			
Pleomorphic astrocytoma		●		
Anaplastic astrocytoma			●	
Glioblastoma				●
Oligodendroglioma		●	● (Anaplastic)	
Ependymoma		●	● (Anaplastic)	
Choroid plexus papilloma	●	● (Atypical)		
Choroid plexus carcinoma			●	
Pineocytoma	●			
Pineoblastoma				●
Medulloblastoma				●
CNS primitive neuroectodermal tumour				●
Schwannoma	●			
Neurofibroma	●			
Malignant peripheral nerve sheath tumour		●	●	●
Meningioma	●	● (Atypical)	● (Anaplastic)	
Craniopharyngioma	●			

b. FALSE – Mostly affect children and/or young adults but they are curable by resection. For this reason pilocytic astrocytomas are classified as grade I. They are most frequently located in the cerebellum, hypothalamus or optic nerve.

c. TRUE – Ependymal cells are epithelial-like cells that line the ventricular system and spinal cord. Hence, ependymomas (a type of glioma) can be commonly found in the spinal cord in adults and posterior fossa in children.

d. TRUE – They generally arise from arachnoid cells (note that pia mater, dura mater and arachnoid form the meninges) and can be intracranial or spinal. They tend to affect patients later into their adulthood, and females are more affected than males. Neurofibromatosis type 2 is associated with a higher risk of meningioma. They are well-defined enhancing lesions.

e. FALSE – They are usually high-grade B-cell lymphomas, strongly enhancing, and commonly found paraventricularly.

A4

Correct answer is A – An alkylating agent that cross-links DNA

The MRI and biopsy findings are highly suggestive of GBM. GBM (WHO grade IV astrocytoma) is the most common *primary* brain tumour in adults and has the worst prognosis.[10] The treatment of GBM is multimodal often involving surgical resection, rotational chemotherapy and/or radiotherapy. Carmustine is a chemotherapeutic drug that has been used to treat GBM. It is an alkylating agent that is bioactivated when it crosses the blood–brain barrier in the CNS. It cross-links DNA, therefore preventing proliferation of tumour cells. Side effects include dizziness and ataxia.

An antibiotic that intercalates DNA (answer B) could be dactinomycin, doxorubicin or bleomycin. Antitumour antibiotics are not indicated for specific use in brain tumours.

An anti-metabolite that decreases DNA synthesis (answer C) could be methotrexate, 5-fluorouracil or 6-mercaptopurine. None of these drugs is indicated for use in brain tumours.

A vinca alkaloid that inhibits microtubule formation (answer D) could be vincristine or vinblastine. Neither of these drugs is indicated for use in brain tumours.

A monoclonal antibody directed against a specific tumour cell receptor (answer E) could include trastuzumab or rituximab. These drugs are not indicated for use in brain tumours.[11]

A⁵

a. iv – An oligodendroglioma is a slow-growing, relatively rare tumour that is most often found in the frontal lobes. It is characterised by a 'fried egg' appearance on histology consisting of round nuclei with a clear cytoplasm. These can calcify. It is important to know the characteristic pathological features of primary CNS tumours, as all tumours can present with non-specific signs such as seizures, confusion and focal lesions.

b. x – Metastatic tumours to the brain are identified as multiple, well-circumscribed tumours commonly found at the grey–white matter junction. In this case, the primary tumour should be vigorously investigated for and found. Primary tumours that metastasise to the brain include tumours from the lung, breast, skin (melanoma) and kidney (renal cell carcinoma).

c. i – GBM is the most common primary brain tumour in adults. It has the worst prognosis and findings indicate a large mass of 'pseudo-palisading' tumour cells that border a central area of necrosis and haemorrhage.

d. iii – Schwannomas are the third most common primary brain tumours in adults. The tumour marker, S-100, is an important marker for schwannomas. It is often localised to the vestibulocochlear nerve (cranial nerve VIII) at the cerebellopontine angle, in which case it is called a vestibular schwannoma or acoustic neuroma. In some cases, a schwannoma may be localised to the facial nerve (cranial nerve VII). Bilateral acoustic schwannomas can be found in neurofibromatosis type 2.[10]

e. viii – Craniopharyngiomas originate from parts of Rathke's pouch that can compress the optic chiasm from above. This initially causes a bitemporal inferior quadrantanopia, although it can progress to a bitemporal hemianopia. Pituitary adenomas initially compress the optic chiasm from below thereby causing a bitemporal superior quadrantanopia and eventually a bitemporal hemianopia if left untreated. Craniopharyngiomas are the most common childhood supratentorial tumours. It is a benign childhood tumour that can cause over- or underproduction of pituitary hormones. A transphenoidal surgical approach is often needed to excise the tumour.[12]

References

1. Gerrard GE, Franks KN. Overview of the diagnosis and management of brain, spine, and meningeal metastases. *J Neurol Neurosurg Psychiatry*. 2004; **75**(Suppl. 2): ii37–42.

2. McKinney PA. Brain tumours: incidence, survival, and aetiology. *J Neurol Neurosurg Psychiatry*. 2004; **75**(Suppl. 2): ii12–17.

3. Grant R. Overview: brain tumour diagnosis and management. Royal College of Physicians guidelines. *J Neurol Neurosurg Psychiatry*. 2004; **75**(Suppl. 2): ii18–23.

4. DeAngelis LM. Brain tumours. *N Engl J Med*. 2001; **344**(2): 114–23.

5. Collins VP. Brain tumours: classification and genes. *J Neurol Neurosurg Psychiatry*. 2004; **75**(Suppl. 2): ii2–11.

6. Raizer JJ, Abrey LE, editors. *Brain Metastases*. New York, NY: Springer; 2007.

7. Madajewicz S, Karakousis C, West CR, *et al.* Malignant melanoma brain metastases: review of Roswell Park Memorial Institute experience. *Cancer*. 1984; **53**(11): 2550–2.

8. National Institute for Health and Care Excellence. *Improving Outcomes for People with Brain and Other CNS Tumours: the manual*. London: NICE; 2006. Available at: www.nice.org.uk/nicemedia/pdf/CSG_brain_manual.pdf (accessed 25 June 2013).

9. Louis DN, Ohgaki H, Wiestler OD, *et al.* The 2007 WHO classification of tumours of the central nervous system. *Acta Neuropathol*. 2007; **114**(2): 97–109.

10. Frosch MP, Anthony DC, De Girolami U. The central nervous system. In: Kumar V, Abbas AK, Fausto N, *et al. Robbins and Cotran Pathologic Basis of Disease, Professional Edition*. 8th ed. Philadelphia, PA: Saunders Elsevier; 2010. pp. 1330–1.

11. Rang HP, Dale MM, Ritter JM, *et al.* Cancer chemotherapy. *Rang and Dale's Pharmacology*. 6th ed. New York, NY: Churchill Livingstone; 2007. pp. 723–4.

12. Zada G, Lin N, Ojerholm E, *et al.* Craniopharyngioma and other cystic epithelial lesions of the sellar region: a review of clinical, imaging, and histopathological relationships. *Neurosurg Focus*. 2010; **28**(4): E4.

4
Cranial nerves

Q1 A 75-year-old gentleman presented to the GP with diplopia. He is currently being investigated for a lung carcinoma. On examination, he was found to have horizontal diplopia and a convergent squint of the right eye.

Please select the most suitable cranial nerve palsy from the following list.

a. Cranial nerve V palsy
b. Cranial nerve II palsy
c. Cranial nerve IV palsy
d. Cranial nerve VI palsy
e. Cranial nerve III palsy

Q2

   i. Right-sided monocular blindness

  ii. Left-sided monocular blindness

 iii. Bitemporal hemianopia

 iv. Binasal hemianopia

  v. Right homonymous hemianopia

 vi. Left homonymous hemianopia

 vii. Right homonymous superior quadrantanopia

viii. Left homonymous superior quadrantanopia

 ix. Right homonymous inferior quadrantanopia

  x. Left homonymous inferior quadrantanopia

 xi. Right homonymous hemianopia with macula sparing

 xii. Left homonymous hemianopia with macula sparing

Choose the most accurate visual field defect for each of the following visual pathway lesions described.

a. Lesion in the left Meyer's loop

b. Pituitary adenoma compressing the optic chiasm

c. Dissection of the right optic tract

d. Glioblastoma of the occipital lobe affecting the left primary visual cortex

e. Severe optic neuritis of the left eye

Q3 Regarding clinical abnormalities of the pupils, which of the following are true and which are false?

a. Horner's syndrome is caused by a lesion to the parasympathetic pathway and causes a unilateral constricted pupil with associated ptosis.

b. In a relative afferent pupillary defect (RAPD), the consensual light reflex is weaker than the direct light reflex.

c. Argyll Robertson pupils are small, accommodate to near objects but are unreactive to light.

d. Denervation of the ciliary ganglion can lead to a dilated pupil that reacts slowly to bright light.

e. The Edinger–Westphal nucleus responsible for pupillary constriction is located in the midbrain at the level of the superior cerebellar peduncle.

Q4

   i.   Olfactory
  ii.   Optic
 iii.   Oculomotor
  iv.   Trochlear
   v.   Trigeminal
  vi.   Abducens
 vii.   Facial
viii.   Vestibulocochlear
  ix.   Glossopharyngeal
   x.   Vagus
  xi.   Accessory
 xii.   Hypoglossal

The following patients presented with cranial nerve lesions; please select the most appropriate nerve affected. Each option can be used once, more than once, or not at all.

a. A 31-year-old man who had an impaired corneal reflex of the right side of his face but could still raise both his eyebrows, close both eyes fully and smile normally.

b. A 43-year-old woman who has had weakness and a droop on the left side of her face, including an inability to crinkle her forehead, since yesterday.

c. A 36-year-old man has signs of tongue atrophy with fasciculation, weakness in speaking and swallowing. You tested his gag reflex, which was negative bilaterally. He cannot shrug his shoulders and has reduced strength in his trapezius muscles. The efferent pathway of which nerve initiates the gag reflex?

d. A 66-year-old man comes in with a painful, blistering skin rash covering his face in almost a clear line, up to the midpoint of his face. He remembers having chicken pox as a child. He has not travelled anywhere recently but remembers having a mild fever the week before.

e. This cranial nerve passes through the cribriform plate.

Q5 A 46-year-old man with a previous episode of Lyme disease diagnosed a month ago presents with Bell's palsy caused by *Borrelia burgdorferi*. What nerve is affected in Bell's palsy?

a. Mandibular
b. Facial
c. Ophthalmic
d. Maxillary
e. Vagus

Answers

A¹

Correct answer is D – Cranial nerve VI palsy

In this case the patient has a right-sided cranial nerve VI palsy, which means the right eye is subjected to unopposed action from the medial rectus muscle causing a convergent squint and hence a horizontal diplopia.

The key piece of information in the history is the patient is being investigated for lung cancer. This means there is a significant chance the patient may have cranial metastases that can result in an increased ICP. Since the course of cranial nerve VI is straight and anterior from the brainstem, if the brainstem is pushed backwards, it will often damage cranial nerve VI by stretching it. This would mean that even though there is a cranial nerve VI palsy, and one would expect an anatomical lesion of cranial nerve VI, the actual pathology is the raised ICP pushing the brainstem backwards causing indirect damage to cranial nerve VI. This is known as a false localising sign – that is, the anatomical location of pathology is not that which is expected.

Increased ICP can be caused by supratentorial or infratentorial space-occupying lesions, idiopathic intracranial hypertension or cerebral venous sinus thrombosis.[1]

A²

a. vii – Right homonymous superior quadrantanopia. Meyer's loop carries fibres from the inferior retina but the image is inverted and so the deficit is actually superior. Baum's loop carries fibres from the superior retina and so a lesion here would cause an inferior quadrantanopia.

b. iii – Bitemporal hemianopia. Pituitary adenomas compress the optic chiasm from below and so even though the deficit is a bitemporal hemianopia, the superior temporal quadrants are actually slightly worse than the inferior temporal quadrants. Craniopharyngiomas often compress the chiasm from above and hence the opposite is true, the deficit is slightly greater in the inferior temporal quadrants. Detection of red light is usually first to go and so using a red pin to test visual fields for these patients can be more sensitive. These patients usually have Goldmann visual field tests done before and after pituitary surgery to formally record pre- and post-operative change in vision.

c. vi – Left homonymous hemianopia. A lesion in the right optic tract causes the loss of function of the left nasal retina and the right temporal retina resulting in a loss of vision from the left hemi field (contralateral homonymous hemianopia).

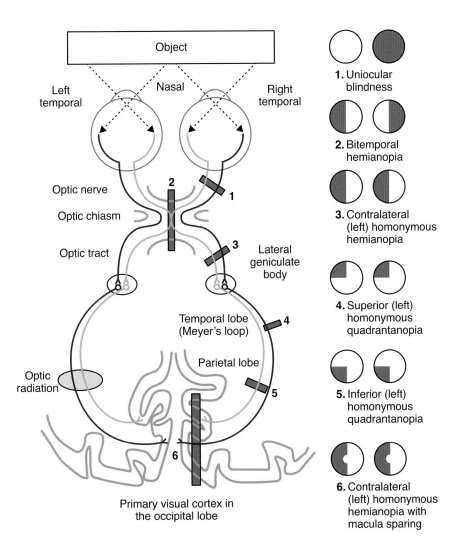

d. xi – Right homonymous hemianopia with macula sparing. In a lesion of the left primary visual cortex, there is a complete visual deficit of the right hemi field but there is macula sparing, most likely because of the extensive representation of the fovea.

e. ii – Left-sided monocular blindness. Optic neuritis is most commonly seen in conditions such as MS, infections (syphilis), systemic lupus erythematosus, vasculitis and diabetes.

A3

a. FALSE – Horner's syndrome is caused by a lesion to the sympathetic pathway and hence the patient may present with a fixed unilateral constricted pupil (unopposed innervation from the Edinger–Westphal nucleus), ptosis, enophthalmos and loss of sweating on the same side of the face or body.
- 'MAPLE': **M**iosis, **A**nhydrosis, **P**tosis, **L**oss of ciliospinal reflex and **E**nophthalmos
- Causes include cerebral infarction, syringomyelia, apical tumours of the bronchus, trauma to the brachial plexus, and after dissection of the neck (e.g. thyroidectomy).[2]

b. FALSE – In a RAPD, the consensual light reflex is stronger than the direct. In a left eye affected by optic neuritis, to test for a RAPD:
1. shine light into the left eye – there should be constriction in both pupils
2. shine light into the right eye – both pupils should again constrict
3. now, shine light into the left eye again and it should dilate.

c. TRUE – This sign is almost diagnostic of neurosyphilis.

d. TRUE – Myotonic pupil (also known as Holmes-Adie pupil) occurs when there is degeneration of the ciliary ganglion. It is usually seen in women and is associated with reduced tendon reflexes.

e. FALSE – The Edinger–Westphal nucleus is actually located in the midbrain at the level of the superior colliculus.

A4

a. v – Trigeminal. The nasocilliary branch of the ophthalmic division (V_1) of the trigeminal nerve carries sensory afferent fibres from the cornea. The facial nerve (cranial nerve VII) initiates the motor response to blink when the nasocilliary branches of V_1 are activated. This forms the blink reflex. The patient in the question has an intact facial nerve on examination; therefore there must be a lesion of the trigeminal nerve.

b. vii – Facial. The woman is presenting with a lower motor neurone lesion of her facial nerve. If the lesion was upper motor neurone, then there would be forehead sparing, so the patient would still be able to raise her left eyebrow. She may also demonstrate other signs, such as hyperacusis or oversensitivity to certain sounds (cranial nerve VII innervates the stapedius) and she may lose taste in the anterior two-thirds of the tongue.

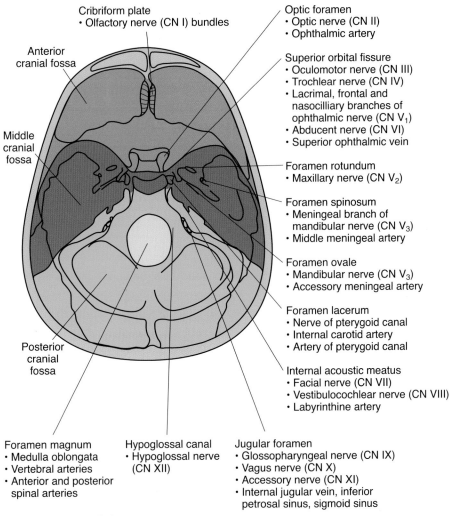

Cribriform plate
• Olfactory nerve (CN I) bundles

Optic foramen
• Optic nerve (CN II)
• Ophthalmic artery

Anterior
cranial fossa

Superior orbital fissure
• Oculomotor nerve (CN III)
• Trochlear nerve (CN IV)
• Lacrimal, frontal and nasocilliary branches of ophthalmic nerve (CN V_1)
• Abducent nerve (CN VI)
• Superior ophthalmic vein

Middle
cranial
fossa

Foramen rotundum
• Maxillary nerve (CN V_2)

Foramen spinosum
• Meningeal branch of mandibular nerve (CN V_3)
• Middle meningeal artery

Foramen ovale
• Mandibular nerve (CN V_3)
• Accessory meningeal artery

Foramen lacerum
• Nerve of pterygoid canal
• Internal carotid artery
• Artery of pterygoid canal

Posterior
cranial
fossa

Internal acoustic meatus
• Facial nerve (CN VII)
• Vestibulocochlear nerve (CN VIII)
• Labyrinthine artery

Foramen magnum
• Medulla oblongata
• Vertebral arteries
• Anterior and posterior spinal arteries

Hypoglossal canal
• Hypoglossal nerve (CN XII)

Jugular foramen
• Glossopharyngeal nerve (CN IX)
• Vagus nerve (CN X)
• Accessory nerve (CN XI)
• Internal jugular vein, inferior petrosal sinus, sigmoid sinus

Key: cranial nerve (CN)

c. x – Vagus. These are signs of bulbar palsy, so called as it affects cranial nerves IX–XII at the level of the medulla. Hence, this affects the lower motor neurones. Pseudobulbar palsy affects the same cranial nerves although the lesion is at the level of the corticobulbar tracts at the mid-pons and therefore the patient experiences upper motor neurone signs (e.g. spastic tongue and brisk jaw reflexes).

d. v – Trigeminal. Shingles, reactivation of the varicella zoster virus dormant in the dorsal root ganglion, causing a painful blistering rash to appear in a dermatomal pattern.

e. i – Olfactory. The cribriform plate is located on the ethmoid bone.[3,4]

A[5]

Correct answer is B – Facial

Bell's palsy is ipsilateral paralysis of the upper and lower face, with inability to close the eye on the involved side. It is the complete destruction of the facial nucleus or its efferent fibres.

It is seen as a complication of Lyme disease, herpes simplex and diabetes mellitus.[3,4]

Some features are highlighted in the mnemonic BELLS Palsy:

- **B**link reflex abnormal
- **E**arache
- **L**acrimation (deficient, excessive)
- **L**oss of taste
- **S**udden onset
- **P**alsy of cranial nerve VII muscles

References

1. Larner AJ. False localising signs. *J Neurol Neurosurg Psychiatry.* 2003; **74**(4): 415–18.
2. George A, Haydar AA, Adams WM. Imaging of Horner's syndrome. *Clin Radiol.* 2008; **63**(5): 499–505.
3. Fitzgerald MJT, Gruener G, Mtui E. *Clinical Neuroanatomy and Neuroscience.* 5th ed. Edinburgh: Elsevier Saunders; 2007.
4. Kumar P, Clark ML, editors. *Kumar & Clark's Clinical Medicine.* 7th ed. Edinburgh: Saunders Elsevier; 2009.

5

Electrophysiology

Q1 A researcher experiments with the nerve conduction velocities of various different nerve types. What would you expect the maximum conduction velocities of the following fibres to be, in order from fastest to slowest?

	Fibre type
A	Alpha motor neurone
B	Sensory A delta fibre
C	Sensory C fibre
D	Gamma motor neurone
E	Preganglionic sympathetic B fibre

a. A, B, D, C, E

b. D, A, B, E, C

c. A, B, D, E, C

d. B, A, D, E, C

e. B, D, A, E, C

Q2 A 5-year-old attended the neurophysiology outpatient clinic after being referred for suspected epilepsy. Electroencephalography (EEG) was performed and a typical 3 Hz spike and wave discharges were seen. What type of epilepsy is commonly associated with these discharges?

a. Frontal lobe seizure

b. Myoclonic seizure

c. Absence seizure

d. Non-epileptic seizure

e. Partial complex seizure

Q3 In patients with definite diagnosis of epilepsy, sleep-deprived EEG has a diagnostic yield of:

a. 25%

b. 35%

c. 50%

d. 75%

e. 95%

Q4 A 55-year-old man, with uncontrolled diabetes mellitus, presented with 6 months' history of numbness in his feet. He underwent nerve conduction studies on his legs. Which are the most likely changes to his sensory conduction?

a. Normal sensory conduction

b. Normal velocity with reduced amplitude

c. Normal velocity with increased amplitude

d. Reduced velocity with reduced amplitude

e. Reduced velocity with normal amplitude

Q5 A 58-year-old woman presents to her GP with an ache in her forearm and hand that is worse at night. She complains of a tingling sensation in her thumb, index and middle fingers. She is otherwise healthy besides a medical history of rheumatoid arthritis. The GP performs Phalen's manoeuvre, which is negative. However, the reverse Phalen's performs is positive. What is the most appropriate investigation in order to diagnose this patient?

a. MRI

b. Serological investigation

c. Nerve conduction studies

d. Electromyography

e. Ultrasound

Answers

A¹

Correct answer is C – A, B, D, E, C

The alpha motor neurone is the fastest mammalian nerve, with a conduction velocity of 70–120 m/s. Sensory A delta fibres have a conduction velocity from 2 to 30 m/s. The gamma motor neurone, which innervates intrafusal muscle fibres has a conduction velocity of 4–24 m/s. Preganglionic sympathetic B fibres have been shown to have a conduction velocity of 6–8 m/s. Lastly, sensory C fibres (non-myelinated) transmitting somatosensory pain have the slowest conduction speed, of around 1.2 m/s.

A²

Correct answer is C – Absence seizure

These are a primary generalised type of seizure. Electroencephalogram changes on their own cannot indicate the diagnosis of epilepsy. However, in absence seizures, the typical 3 Hz spike and wave charges can be seen if the patient has a seizure during the recording. This type of seizure can often be provoked by hyperventilation.[1,2]

A³

Correct answer is D – 75%

The basic electroencephalogram test has a 50% diagnostic yield of patients with definite epilepsy. However, with sleep-deprived EEG, the diagnostic yield increases to 75%. Another technique to increase the EEG diagnostic yield includes forced hyperventilation for 3 minutes.[2]

A4

Correct answer is B – Normal velocity with reduced amplitude

Diabetes mellitus is one of the commonest causes of peripheral neuropathy in developed countries. Nerve conduction studies confirm whether axons, myelin or both of these are affected. However, in diabetes mellitus, axons are damaged with intact myelin sheath. This is the reason why amplitude is mostly affected with velocity being unaffected.[2,3]

A5

Correct answer is C – Nerve conduction studies

This woman is most likely to have carpal tunnel syndrome (CTS). This is evidenced by the paraesthesia in her thumb, index and middle fingers as well as her associated rheumatoid arthritis and the positive reverse Phalen's test.[4] Pain was elicited in the reverse Phalen's test because of the higher intra-carpal tunnel hydrostatic pressure compared with in the normal Phalen's manoeuvre.[5] Other features of median nerve compression on examination include wasting of the thenar eminence, weakness of the lateral two **L**umbricals, **O**pponens pollicis, **A**bductor pollicis brevis and **F**lexor pollicis brevis (remembered by the useful mnemonic 'LOAF', with the thenar eminence involving 'OAF').

Nerve conduction studies in order to measure motor and sensory conduction times are a first-line investigation when CTS is suspected.[6] Ultrasound is being used increasingly to confirm CTS, as it is cheaper and faster, although nerve conduction studies maintain the highest sensitivity and specificity for diagnosis.

References

1. Colledge NR, Walker BR, Ralston SH, editors. *Davidson's Principles and Practice of Medicine*. 21st ed. Edinburgh: Elsevier Science; 2010.
2. Fuller G, Manford M. *Neurology: an illustrated colour text*. Edinburgh: Elsevier; 2010.
3. Haslett C, Chilvers ER, Boon N, editors. *Davidson's Principles and Practice of Medicine*. 19th ed. Edinburgh: Elsevier Science; 2002.
4. Longmore M, Wilkinson IB, Davidson EH, *et al*. *Oxford Handbook of Clinical Medicine*. 8th ed. New York, NY: Oxford University Press; 2010.

5. Werner RA, Bir C, Armstrong TJ. Reverse Phalen's maneuver as an aid in diagnosing carpal tunnel syndrome. *Arch Phys Med Rehabil*. 1994; **75**(7): 783–6.

6. Campbell ED. The carpal tunnel syndrome: investigation and assessment of treatment. *Proc R Soc Med*. 1962; **55**: 401–5.

6

Epilepsy

Q1 Please select the most appropriate anti-epileptic drug (AED) from the following list for each of the following scenarios.

   i. Sodium valproate

  ii. Carbamazepine

 iii. Phenytoin

 iv. Lamotrigine

  v. Gabapentin

 vi. Ethosuximide

 vii. Phenobarbital

viii. Topiramate

a. A 22-year-old female has been experiencing tonic–clonic seizures and wishes to conceive in the near future. What is the AED of choice?

b. A known epileptic patient presents with blurred vision and vertigo. Blood results show hyponatraemia and leucopenia. Select which AED produces these side effects.

c. An 8-year-old girl presents after daydreaming at school. EEG shows characteristic a 3 Hz spike and wave discharges. Select the most suitable AED to start.

d. A 29-year-old male suffers with atonic seizures. Which AED is the first-line treatment?

e. A 25-year-old male has recently started a new medication for myoclonic seizures in conjunction with what he was already on. He presented today with pins and needles in the arms. Which AED can cause paraesthesia?

Q2 Please select the most likely diagnosis from the list below for the following scenarios.

   i. Tonic–clonic seizure
   ii. Clonic seizure
   iii. Atonic seizure
   iv. Temporal lobe epilepsy
   v. Rolandic epilepsy
   vi. West syndrome
   vii. Absence seizure
   viii. Juvenile myoclonic epilepsy

   a. A 7-month-old girl presents with brief axial movements. EEG shows hypsarrhythmia.
   b. A 16-year-old boy presents after his mother witnessed him having a seizure with both arms and legs shaking. On further questioning, she advises that he spills his breakfast in the morning and daydreams frequently at school.
   c. A 23-year-old lady complains of intense feelings of déjà vu and strange sensations in her stomach lasting for 1–2 minutes at a time.
   d. A 6-year-old boy presents to the hospital after his parents noticed a whole-body seizure. On further questioning, the child tells you that his tongue tingled before the seizure.

Q3 In patients presenting with a seizure for the first time, which of the following is an indication for a CT scan of the brain?
   a. Fever
   b. Partial-onset seizures
   c. Transient post-ictal headache
   d. Age over 40 years
   e. Tonic–clonic seizure without aura

Q4 With Lennox–Gastaut syndrome (LGS), which of the following statements are true and which are false?

a. Onset is most often in pre-adolescent children.

b. EEG of these patients usually shows diffuse slow spike and waves of ~2 Hz frequency.

c. The most common seizures experienced in this syndrome are partial.

d. The mortality rate of patients with LGS is less than 2%.

e. LGS can be preceded by a diagnosis of West syndrome.

Q5 A 64-year-old woman presents to the A&E department having suffered a generalised tonic–clonic seizure. One week prior to this event, she also suffered a stroke and as a result is now hemiplegic. Which of the following statements are true and which are false?

a. She has now developed epilepsy as a result of the stroke.

b. The stroke was most likely ischaemic.

c. The National Institute for Health and Care Excellence states that anti-epileptic treatment should only be started after a second seizure.

d. Carbamazepine is a first-generation AED.

e. Glial scarring can lead to epileptogenesis.

Q6 A 20-year-old male was admitted to the A&E department following a fit, witnessed by his girlfriend. Previously, he had a history of an unwitnessed collapse with tongue biting. Which investigation is most appropriately used to diagnose and characterise his epilepsy?

a. CT head

b. MRI head

c. Nerve conduction study

d. EEG

e. Electrocardiogram

Answers

A1

a. iv – Lamotrigine. For generalised tonic–clonic seizures only (no myoclonic seizures and no suspicion of juvenile myoclonic epilepsy), lamotrigine or sodium valproate is usually the first-line treatment. However, in women planning to conceive, it is safer to use lamotrigine rather than sodium valproate, as the latter has a significantly higher risk of teratogenic side effects to the unborn child. The National Institute for Health and Care Excellence recommends that a high-resolution ultrasound scan should be offered to pregnant women on AEDs at 18–20 weeks of gestation and all children born to mothers taking enzyme-inducing AEDs should receive 1 mg of vitamin K at delivery to prevent haemorrhagic disease of the newborn.

b. ii – Carbamazepine. It is usually recommended for focal seizures (can also consider lamotrigine), late-onset occipital epilepsy, trigeminal neuralgia and bipolar disorder unresponsive to lithium. A dose of 100–200 mg is given initially and then slowly increased to minimise the risk of hyponatraemia and leucopenia.

c. vi – Ethosuximide. The typical EEG finding is that seen in patients suffering absence seizures. The first-line treatment is usually ethosuximide. Sodium valproate can be considered if there is a high risk of generalised tonic–clonic seizures as well as absence seizures.

d. i – Sodium valproate. Atonic seizures are generalised seizures characterised by sudden onset of loss of muscle tone. Sodium valproate is usually the first-line treatment; lamotrigine can be given as an adjunct if symptoms are not adequately controlled.

e. viii – Topiramate. It can be given alone or with other medications (adjunct) for generalised tonic–clonic seizures, focal seizures, absence seizures or myoclonic seizures. Dose is increased slowly due to side effects and dosage tailored to whether monotherapy or adjunct.

A²

a. vi – West syndrome. Also known as infantile spasms, there is no gender preponderance, it accounts for 2% of all childhood epilepsies, and presents between 3 and 12 months of age. The child's head will fall towards their feet and then they will suddenly become upright. These are known as 'lightning', 'jack knife' or 'salaam' attacks.

b. viii – Juvenile myoclonic epilepsy. This presents during puberty and most commonly as a triad of myoclonic, tonic–clonic and absence seizures. Also known as Kellogg's seizures, as the seizures are common in the morning. First-line treatment is usually with sodium valproate.

c. iv – Temporal lobe epilepsy. This is a type of focal (partial) epilepsy which can be simple (consciousness maintained) or complex (consciousness impaired). Sensory symptoms include patients experiencing odd smells (olfactory disturbance), hearing strange sounds (auditory disturbance) and having strange sensations in their stomach (gustatory disturbance). Autonomic symptoms include palpitations and sweating. Psychic symptoms include feelings of déjà vu, *jamais vu*, fear, anxiety and depersonalisation. In complex partial seizures, patients may experience impaired consciousness and therefore may stare blankly, experience behavioural arrest or experience automated movements such as lip-smacking, chewing and swallowing. First-line treatment is usually with carbamazepine or lamotrigine.

d. v – Rolandic epilepsy. This accounts for approximately 15% of epilepsy in children, mostly affecting children aged 6–8 years. The seizures start around the somato-motor area of the brain (also known as the Rolandic area) just anterior to the central sulcus of the brain. For this reason, patients can experience unilateral facial symptoms, oropharyngolaryngeal symptoms such as numbness and tingling inside the mouth, anarthria (inability to talk) and hypersalivation.

A3

Correct answer is B – Partial-onset seizures

Partial-onset seizures are an indication for a CT scan because there might be focal organic pathology compared to generalised tonic–clonic seizure without aura. If the patient had a persistent post-ictal headache this would also be a reason to obtain intracranial imaging to exclude a bleed/other organic pathology.

A4

a. FALSE – Onset is usually in children aged 3–10 years. LGS is often difficult to treat and sufferers have frequent and different types of seizures.

b. TRUE

c. FALSE – Most common are general tonic seizures and myoclonic seizures, although partial seizures can also be experienced.

d. FALSE – Ranges from about 3% to 7%.

e. TRUE – West syndrome (also known as infantile spasms) is characterised by symmetrical bilateral flexion/extension seizures involving the neck, trunk, arms and legs. These types of seizures are sometimes referred to as 'salaam' seizures or 'jack knife' seizures. Children with West syndrome tend to 'grow out' of these flexion/extension seizures but invariably go on to develop other types of epileptic seizures and some can develop LGS. Children with LGS tend to have multiple and varied seizure types including atonic, tonic–clonic and absence seizures (previously known as petit-mal seizures).

A5

a. FALSE – Although this lady has suffered an early onset seizure (a seizure that occurs within 2 weeks of a stroke), she cannot be diagnosed with epilepsy on the basis of a single episode. She has an approximately 33% chance of a recurrent seizure and hence an increased risk of developing epilepsy.[1]

b. FALSE – Haemorrhagic stroke is more commonly associated with seizures. Focal ischaemia around the haemorrhage, haemosiderin deposition as a result of phagocytosis of red blood cells and the mass effect of haematomas all contribute to the epileptogenesis of the brain following a haemorrhagic stroke.[2]

c.   FALSE – The guidelines state that even though treatment should be considered mainly after a second unprovoked seizure, it can be considered after a single episode – especially if the patient has a neurological defect.[3]

d.   TRUE – Before 1991 there were 10 drugs licensed for anti-epileptic use including carbamazepine, acetazolamide, clonazepam, ethosuximide, phenytoin and sodium valproate; these are known as first-generation AEDs. Second-generation AEDs such as lamotrigine, gabapentin and levetiracetam were then licensed and shown to be better tolerated and to have a higher efficacy.[4]

e.   TRUE – Astrocytes (a specific type of glial cell) recycle the excitatory neurotransmitter glutamate from the synaptic cleft and if they are damaged this may lead to excito-toxicity and hence an increased risk of seizures.[5]

A[6]

Correct answer is D – EEG

The diagnosis of epilepsy is mainly clinical, although EEG helps in the diagnosis and characterisation of epilepsy. However, if normal, an EEG does not exclude the diagnosis. A CT or MRI of the head can help to investigate for structural abnormalities that EEG cannot be used for.[6]

References

1. Kotila M, Waltimo O. Epilepsy after stroke. *Epilepsia*. 1992; **33**(3): 495–8.
2. Myint PK, Staufenberg EF, Sabanathan K. Post-stroke seizure and post-stroke epilepsy. *Postgrad Med J*. 2006; **82**(971): 568–72.
3. Stokes T, Shaw EJ, Juarez-Garcia A, *et al. Clinical Guidelines and Evidence Review for the Epilepsies: diagnosis and management in adults and children in primary and secondary care.* London: Royal College of General Practitioners; 2004. Available at: www.nice.org.uk/nicemedia/live/10954/29533/29533.pdf (accessed 10 January 2013).

4. Epilepsy Action. *Epilepsy Medicines Available in the United Kingdom*. Leeds: Epilepsy Action; May 2013. Available at: www.epilepsy.org.uk/info/drugslist.html (accessed 26 July 2013).
5. Olsen TS. Post-stroke epilepsy. *Curr Arthroscler Rep*. 2001; **3**(4): 340–4.
6. Fuller G, Manford M. *Neurology: an illustrated colour text*. Edinburgh: Elsevier; 2010.

7

Genetics

$Q1$ A 2-year-old child is brought to the consultant paediatrician because of frequent stumbling and falling. His mother explains that the child had a notable deformed back in his first year. On examination, the child is found to have pes cavus, nystagmus and a staggering gait. On genetic analysis, the child is found to have a trinucleotide repeat disorder of $(GAA)^n$. What is the most likely diagnosis?

a. Tabes dorsalis

b. Friedreich's ataxia

c. Werdnig–Hoffmann disease

d. Binswanger's disease

e. Fragile X syndrome

Q2 A 27-year-old male university student presents with cloudy vision and loss of hair on his head. His GP confirms a cataract in his left eye and frontal baldness. He also notes there is some facial weakness, with wasting of the jaw muscles and temporalis muscles. There is also weakness of the distal limb muscles and myotonia. The patient's father also had a similar but less severe illness that started in his early 40s. The GP suspects a diagnosis of myotonic dystrophy. If a genetic analysis is ordered to confirm this diagnosis, what trinucleotide repeat pattern would be seen?

   a. $(CAG)^n$

   b. $(CTG)^n$

   c. $(CGG)^n$

   d. $(GAA)^n$

   e. $(CGA)^n$

Q3 A 14-year-old girl is referred to the consultant paediatrician because of painful muscle cramps in her legs. Family history demonstrates similar conditions in several generations affecting both sexes. The girl is found to have an unusually high arch in both her feet and clawing of her toes. Her calves look extremely thin and wasted. She has also lost her sense of light touch but she is responsive to painful stimuli. What is the most likely cause of the findings in this young girl?

   a. A trinucleotide repeat disorder in the gene that encodes frataxin

   b. Antibody-mediated destruction of beta cells in the pancreas

   c. A mutation in the gene that encodes dystrophin

   d. Autoimmune inflammation and demyelination

   e. Defective production of proteins involved in the structure and function of myelin

Q4 Which of the following statements are true and which are false?

a. Becker's muscular dystrophy is associated with the DMD gene.

b. Huntington's disease (HD) is an autosomal dominant, trinucleotide repeat disorder of 'GAC'.

c. von Recklinghausen's disease is a neuro-ectodermal syndrome associated with neurofibromatosis type 2.

d. Friedreich's ataxia is an autosomal dominant, trinucleotide repeat disorder of 'GAA'.

e. Amyotrophic lateral sclerosis (ALS) is associated with a defect in superoxide dismutase 1 and is progressive and fatal.

Answers

A1

Correct answer is B – Friedreich's ataxia

Friedreich's ataxia is a trinucleotide repeat disorder of $(GAA)^n$ in the gene that encodes frataxin. This condition displays an autosomal recessive pattern of inheritance and hence genetic anticipation is not observed since the disease is typically not observed in more than one generation (unlike HD in which there is genetic anticipation as there is an autosomal dominant pattern of inheritance).

Symptoms usually begin in childhood, characterised by a slowly progressive ataxia and associated with weakness, scoliosis, bladder dysfunction, hypo/a-reflexia, dysarthria. Demyelination of the dorsal columns can also cause loss of proprioception and vibration sense. Cardiomyopathy and diabetes are also commonly associated with Friedreich's ataxia.[1]

Tabes dorsalis (answer A) is characteristic of tertiary syphilis. Degeneration of the dorsal columns and dorsal roots results in ataxia. Proprioception, vibration and discriminatory touch are affected.

Werdnig–Hoffmann disease (answer C) is also known as spinal muscular atrophy type 1 (SMA1). It is an autosomal recessive condition that leads to degeneration of anterior horn cells resulting in muscle weakness and wasting. It characteristically affects those aged less than 6 months and hence it can present as 'floppy baby'.

Binswanger's disease (answer D) is a small vessel vascular dementia that results in memory loss and decline in cognitive ability. White matter lesions are thought to occur due to atherosclerosis. It usually presents in older persons.

Fragile X syndrome (answer E), also known as Martin–Bell syndrome, is a trinucleotide repeat disorder of $(CGG)^n$. It is the second most common cause of genetic mental retardation after Down's syndrome. Patients have an elongated face, large or protruding ears, pes planus, macro-orchidism and hypotonia.

A²

Correct answer is B – $(CTG)^n$

Myotonic dystrophy is a disease that affects skeletal and smooth muscle as well as multiple other organ systems. There is myotonic dystrophy type 1 (DM1) and type 2. DM1 can be categorised into three overlapping phenotypes: mild, classic and congenital. The patient in this question is likely to have classic DM1 since he has cataracts, myotonia and muscle weakness. Patients can also have cardiac abnormalities and endocrine changes. Congenital DM1 is usually characterised by severe muscle weakness and hypotonia at birth which can often lead to respiratory complications and mortality. It displays an autosomal dominant inheritance pattern and genetic anticipation.[2] Genetic anticipation is the concept that a worsening severity of disease or an earlier onset of disease is evident in succeeding generations. This is because succeeding generations display a longer trinucleotide repeat sequence than their predecessors. Other trinucleotide repeat disorders include HD and fragile X syndrome.[3]

   $(CAG)^n$ (answer A) is a trinucleotide repeat pattern seen in HD.

   $(CGG)^n$ (answer C) is a trinucleotide repeat pattern seen in fragile X syndrome.

   $(GAA)^n$ (answer D) is a trinucleotide repeat pattern seen in Friedreich's ataxia.

   $(CGA)^n$ (answer E) is a trinucleotide repeat pattern not linked to any disease.

A³

Correct answer is E – Defective production of proteins involved in the structure and function of myelin

The findings are highly suggestive of Charcot–Marie–Tooth disease which is a peripheral neuropathy characterised by distal muscle weakness and atrophy, sensory disturbance, hypo/a-reflexia and high-arched feet. It can be inherited in an autosomal dominant, recessive or X-linked pattern depending on the subtype. Management is usually symptomatic with analgesia and involves a multidisciplinary team approach including orthopaedic surgeons for correction of severe pes cavus deformities. Diagnosis can be made through symptoms, electromyography and/or DNA testing/nerve biopsy.[4]

A trinucleotide repeat disorder in the gene that encodes frataxin (answer A) suggests Friedreich's ataxia.

Antibody-mediated destruction of beta cells in the pancreas (answer B) suggests type 1 diabetes mellitus.

A mutation in the gene that encodes dystrophin (answer C) is indicative of Duchenne or Becker's muscular dystrophy.

Autoimmune inflammation and demyelination (answer D) are suggestive of MS.

A4

a. TRUE – Both Becker's and Duchenne muscular dystrophy are X-linked recessive inherited diseases that have genetic mutations of the dystrophin (DMD) gene. In Duchenne muscular dystrophy, there is usually no production of functional dystrophin and hence there is a more severe loss of muscle fibres and greater severity of symptoms. Onset of Becker's is in adolescence whereas in Duchenne onset is commonly in early childhood.[5]

> Remember: Duchenne – **D**eleted **M**uscle **D**ystrophin (DMD gene)

b. FALSE – HD is due to an autosomal dominant trinucleotide 'CAG' repeat disorder. The disease is characterised by chorea, cognitive impairment and psychological disturbance. Atrophy of striatal nuclei may be seen on imaging.[6]

> Remember: 'CAG' repeats – '**C**audate loses **ACh** and **G**amma-Aminobutyric acid (GABA)'

c. FALSE – von Recklinghausen's disease is associated with neurofibromatosis type 1. The disease leads to café au lait spots, Lisch nodules and neural tumours. It has an association with scoliosis.[5]

d. FALSE – Friedreich's ataxia is an autosomal recessive, trinucleotide repeat disorder of 'GAA' in the gene encoding frataxin (a mitochondrial protein). Deficiency in frataxin leads to frequent falls, staggering gait, nystagmus, dysarthria and hammer toes. The cause of death in these patients is usually cardiomyopathy.

e. TRUE – ALS (or Lou Gehrig's disease) is a type of motor neurone disease (MND) associated with both upper and lower motor neurone signs, with no other deficits. Riluzole treatment can lengthen survival in some patients but the disease is progressive and fatal.[5,7]

References

1. Bidichandani SI, Delatycki MB. *Friedreich Ataxia*. 1998 Dec 18 [Updated 2012 Feb 2]. In: Pagon RA, Adam MP, Bird TD, *et al.*, editors. GeneReviews™ [Internet]. Seattle, WA: University of Washington, Seattle; 1993–2013. Available at: www.ncbi.nlm.nih.gov/books/NBK1281/ (accessed 10 January 2013).
2. Bird TD. *Myotonic Dystrophy Type 1*. 1999 Sep 17 [Updated 2013 May 16]. In: Pagon RA, Adam MP, Bird TD, *et al.*, editors. GeneReviews™ [Internet]. Seattle, WA: University of Washington, Seattle; 1993–2013. Available at: www.ncbi.nlm. nih.gov/books/NBK1165/ (accessed 10 January 2013).
3. Kumar V, Abbas AK, Fausto N, *et al*. Genetic disorders. *Robbins and Cotran Pathologic Basis of Disease, Professional Edition*. 8th ed. Philadelphia, PA: Saunders Elsevier; 2010. p. 168.
4. Pareyson D, Marchesi C. Diagnosis, natural history, and management of Charcot–Marie–Tooth disease. *Lancet Neurol*. 2009; **8**(7): 654–67.
5. Kumar P, Clark ML, editors. *Kumar & Clark's Clinical Medicine*. 7th ed. Edinburgh: Saunders Elsevier; 2009.
6. Goljan EF. *Rapid Review Pathology*. 3rd ed. Philadelphia, PA: Mosby/Elsevier; 2010.
7. MedlinePlus. *Amyotrophic Lateral Sclerosis*. Bethesda, MD: US National Library of Medicine; 2012. Available at: www.nlm.nih.gov/medlineplus/amyotrophiclateral sclerosis.html (accessed 10 January 2013).

8

Intracranial haemorrhage

Q1 A 58-year-old man presents with a 3-day history of worsening head-ache and nausea. His medical history is unremarkable besides chronic alcohol abuse and you discover that he was assaulted 1 week ago. His blood pressure is 108/84 mmHg, heart rate 85 bpm, respiratory rate 16 breaths per minute and temperature 36.7°C. The patient appears to be confused.

Investigations:
- haemoglobin 13.7 g/dL (13.5–17.5 g/dL)
- white blood count 10.3 × 10⁹/L (4–11 × 10⁹/L)
- neutrophils 6.4 × 10⁹/L (2.0–7.5 × 10⁹/L)
- sodium 136 mmol/L (135–146 mmol/L)

The most likely diagnosis is:
a. Intraparenchymal haemorrhage
b. Extradural haemorrhage
c. Intraventricular haemorrhage
d. SAH
e. Subdural haematoma

Q2

   i. Re-bleed

   ii. Hyponatraemia

   iii. Vasodilation

   iv. Hydrocephalus

   v. Vasospasm

   vi. Hypernatraemia

   vii. Seizures

Regarding aneurysmal SAH:

a. Which of these listed complications leads to the worst prognosis?

b. Which of these listed complications may cause a delayed ischaemic neurological deficit (DIND)?

c. For which of these listed complications may a CSF diversion procedure be appropriate?

d. Which of these listed complications must be corrected slowly?

Q3

A 79-year-old man who takes warfarin for atrial fibrillation is brought to his GP with a gradual onset of confusion and left-sided weakness, worsening over the previous 3 weeks. On close questioning, the patient advises he fell 4 weeks prior to presentation and bruised his forehead but had no neurological problems at that time. What is the most likely diagnosis?

a. Ischaemic stroke

b. CNS tumour

c. Chronic subdural haematoma (CSDH)

d. SAH

Q4

Regarding CSDHs, which of the following may be appropriate management strategies?

a. Burr hole evacuation of the haematoma

b. Craniotomy and evacuation of the haematoma

c. Observation with neurological examinations and repeat CT scans

d. All of the above

Q5 With regard to traumatic brain injury, which of the following statements are true and which are false?

a. A middle meningeal artery tear is often the cause of a subdural haemorrhage.

b. Subdural haematomas are venous in origin.

c. Lumbar puncture is usually the first-line diagnostic tool in patients with suspected SAHs.

d. SAHs are most commonly seen in patients with an Arnold–Chiari malformation.

e. With severe traumatic brain injury, decorticate posturing where the arms are extended to the side, and decerebrate posturing with the arms flexed over the chest can be seen.

Answers

A¹

Correct answer is E – Subdural haematoma

The history of a 3-day worsening headache suggests a slow venous bleed in keeping with an acute subdural haematoma. SAHs are usually due to burst berry aneurysms (in non-trauma patients) and present with sudden-onset 'thunderclap' headaches (usually occipital and associated with vomiting and meningism). An extradural haemorrhage is usually caused by rupture of the middle meningeal artery from direct trauma to the side of the skull. In this case however, the patient deteriorated over 3 days, whereas if it was an extradural haemorrhage, it would bleed much faster and cause more severe symptoms rapidly.[1]

Subdural haematomas can be acute (<3 days), subacute (3–21 days) or chronic (>21 days). They usually have different aetiologies depending on age: in children always suspect non-accidental injury, in young adults they are usually due to trauma (e.g. road traffic accident) and in older persons usually because of falls (older individuals are more susceptible since they have increased brain atrophy).[2]

A²

a. i – Recurrent haemorrhage is a well reported phenomenon following a SAH. Studies suggest most re-bleeds occur on the first day and carry a dismal prognosis with fatality rates around 70%. Delayed admission to hospital from initial SAH symptom onset, high blood pressure, poor neurological status on admission and insertion of ventriculostomy drains post-operatively are all associated with increased rates of re-bleeding.[3]

b. v – Vasospasm. Cerebral vasospasm is delayed narrowing of cerebral vessels following a SAH. It normally begins 3 days after the haemorrhage with a peak at 5–14 days. It can cause reduced distal blood flow and can lead to DIND and cerebral infarction if left untreated. It is worth noting that vasospasm on angiography does not necessarily always correlate with clinical symptoms of vasospasm.[3]

c. iv – Hydrocephalus. CSF diversion is recommended for patients with ventriculomegaly and reduced level of consciousness after SAH via ventriculostomy, and permanent shunting may be required in symptomatic patients with chronic hydrocephalus.[3]

d. ii – Hyponatraemia. Rapid correction of hyponatraemia can lead to central pontine myelinolysis, a condition involving demyelination predominantly of the basis pontis. This is due to osmotic changes as a result of alterations in sodium concentration. It is rare, especially in acute hyponatraemia; however, it is a recognised complication. It may cause 'locked-in' syndrome. Extrapontine myelinolysis is the same disease process but in different anatomical sites and therefore presents differently.[4]

A³

Correct answer is C – CSDH

These symptoms fit best with a CSDH because of the progressive and insidious nature of the symptoms, and is more likely due to the history of minor trauma and being on warfarin. A subdural haematoma is caused by rupture of bridging veins, and the haematoma becomes encapsulated. The haematoma may then resolve as it is resorbed, or it may enlarge as a CSDH. The growth of the CSDH is thought to be due to recurrent bleeding from abnormal, dilated blood vessels in the haematoma capsule. Because of age-related atrophy, it can take some time before symptoms develop.[5]

A⁴

Correct answer is D – All of the above

Depending on the size of the CSDH and clinical condition of the patient, all of the listed strategies may be appropriate. Burr hole evacuation of the haematoma may be possible but in larger subacute haematomas craniotomy may be necessary, or it may be necessary for patients with re-accumulation of the blood following surgery. If the CSDH is small, it may be resorbed spontaneously, and in this case the patient must be monitored carefully for clinical deterioration.[5]

A5

a. FALSE – This is classically an extradural haemorrhage as a result of a blow to the side of the head over the pterion region (where the middle meningeal artery lies).

b. TRUE – Rupture of veins traversing the subdural space by shearing forces of excessive movement can lead to subdural haematomas.

c. FALSE – In traumatic brain injury, a CT scan would be performed in the first instance to investigate low Glasgow Coma Scale score/focal neurology/seizures resulting from the injury. Sometimes traumatic subarachnoid blood can be seen on the scan; if this is the case a lumbar puncture or CT angiogram is not required as this is unlikely to have an aneurysmal cause. However, if the subarachnoid blood is in a suspicious area on the scan or the history suggests a collapse before the head injury, a CT angiogram may be warranted to exclude an underlying aneurysm. In patients with non-traumatic SAH, if the initial CT scan is negative then a lumbar puncture is warranted to look for xanthochromia (breakdown products of red blood cells from the subarachnoid blood) and to exclude SAH.

d. FALSE – Arnold–Chiari malformation is usually congenital and results from cerebellar tonsillar descent below the foramen magnum. Non-traumatic SAH is most commonly associated with the rupture of berry aneurysms.

e. FALSE – Decerebrate posturing is arms extended and decorticate is arms flexed. This abnormal posturing is an ominous sign and requires immediate medical attention since it may be a sign that coning of the brain is occurring or about to take place.

References

1. van Gijn J, Kerr RS, Rinkel GJ. Subarachnoid haemorrhage. *Lancet*. 2007; **369**(9558): 306–18.
2. Longmore M, Wilkinson IB, Davidson EH, *et al*. *Oxford Handbook of Clinical Medicine*. 8th ed. New York, NY: Oxford University Press; 2010.
3. Bederson JB, Connolly ES Jr, Batjer HH, *et al*. Guidelines for the management of aneurysmal subarachnoid hemorrhage: a statement for healthcare professionals

from a special writing group of the Stroke Council, American Heart Association. *Stroke.* 2009; **40**(3): 994–1025.

4. Martin RJ. Central pontine and extrapontine myelinolysis: the osmotic demyelination syndromes. *J Neurol Neurosurg Psychiatry.* 2004; **75**(Suppl. 3): iii22–8.

5. Adhiyaman V, Asghar M, Ganeshram KN, *et al.* Chronic subdural haematoma in the elderly. *Postgrad Med J.* 2002; **78**(916): 71–5.

9

Miscellaneous

Q¹

  i. Migraine
 ii. Tension headache
iii. Cervical spondylosis
 iv. Space-occupying lesion
  v. Stress
 vi. Cluster headache
vii. SAH
viii. Sinusitis
 ix. Meningitis

For the following questions, please choose from the answers listed above; the answers may be used once, more than once or not at all. What is the most accurate diagnosis in each patient?

a. A 19-year-old woman complains of severe headaches, described as unilateral, progressively more painful and lasting hours. She noticed flashes of light before the headache started. She has had a lot of work to do recently and this is her second headache in the last 2 months.

b. A 22-year-old student comes in saying she has had a 'band-like pain around her head', almost as if she was wearing a tight headband. She says nothing aggravates it, but she does feel it comes on when she is trying to finish her work late at night.

c. A 20-year-old medical student has been feeling tired and is worried because it has disrupted her revision. She finally sees her GP after a bout of diarrhoea that came with a severe frontal headache over the last day. The headache is 10/10 in terms of pain and is worsened by moving her neck. She does not have an aura but she has been quite withdrawn because loud noises and bright lights aggravate her symptoms.

d. A 25-year-old businessman presents with a short episode of severe unilateral pain. The pain is periorbital and he says it feels like it lasts for hours, during which he can not do anything. He says, 'I'm sweating, my eyes are tearing and I've got this searing pain behind my eye, doctor'. He says he has had this before but he wants somebody to tell him what it is now.

e. A 70-year-old woman presents with a 4-month history of occipital headaches that occasionally radiate to the temporal area. She has been finding it difficult to drive because whenever she turns her head she has stiffness and pain in her neck and shoulders.

Q2

i. Duchenne muscular dystrophy
ii. MG
iii. Denervation atrophy
iv. Nemaline myopathy
v. Facioscapulohumeral muscular dystrophy
vi. Disuse atrophy
vii. Limb-girdle dystrophy
viii. Mitochondrial myopathy
ix. Myotonic dystrophy

Select the most likely diagnosis from the provided list associated with its histopathological finding.

a. Tangles of small rod-shaped granules in type I fibres.
b. Ragged red appearance of muscle fibres.
c. Fibre-type grouping in contrast to the mixture of type I and type II fibres seen in normal muscle.
d. Random variation in muscle fibre size and replacement of necrotic fibres by fibrofatty tissue.
e. Angular atrophy of type II muscle fibres.

Q3 A 57-year-old man presents with a rapidly progressive dementia over a number of months. His wife reports his personality has changed and that he has problems with his gait and balance. Only 2 months later, the man subsequently dies from a severe community-acquired pneumonia. Brain biopsy reveals a spongiform appearance. There are multiple cysts with an absence of inflammatory cells in the grey matter area of the brain. What disease is likely to have killed this patient?

a. Parkinson's disease

b. HD

c. Pick's disease

d. Alzheimer's dementia

e. Creutzfeldt–Jakob disease

Answers

A¹

a. i – The patient describes a classical migraine that is unilateral with an aura. Typically they last 4 to 72 hours and can be associated with nausea or vomiting. Light, noise and physical activity can aggravate the symptoms. Well-known triggers include red wine, chocolate and cheese. Treatment is usually symptomatic relief with simple analgesics such as paracetamol or non-steroidal anti-inflammatory drugs. Triptans are also used in patients who do not respond to simple analgesia.[1]

b. ii – This is the typical pattern of a tension headache. It is brought on by fatigue and stress. Tension headaches are typically bilateral, and described as a tight, band-like pain or pressure around the head. The course of the headache is unpredictable.[1]

c. ix – The associated symptoms of diarrhoea, location of the headache and neck stiffness are strongly suggestive of meningitis. We cannot tell the aetiology from history alone, as we would need a lumbar puncture and CSF culture to reveal this. Kernig's and Brudzinski's signs could also be incorporated into the clinical examination to support the diagnosis.[1,2]

d. vi – These typically occur in males, the average age of onset being 25 years. Presenting with brief episodes of periorbital, excruciating pain that can last anywhere between 30 minutes and 3 hours. The sudden onset of cluster headaches can be easily confused with the more dangerous differential of SAH and should be kept in mind as such. Attacks happen in 'clusters' affecting the same part of the head at the same time of day and are associated with ipsilateral lacrimation of the eye.[1]

e. iii – Cervical spondylosis is a degenerative osteoarthritis of the cervical spine, frequently presenting with occipital headaches that are exacerbated by movement of the neck. These often radiate to the temporal region. If the facet joint osteoarthritis is severe, then nerve root entrapment can occur leading to neurological symptoms such as pain, paraesthesia, numbness and weakness in the upper limbs. In severe cervical spondylosis, the C6 and C7 nerve roots are commonly affected.[3] Always keep in mind the diagnosis of giant cell arteritis (GCA) in patients presenting with headache in the temporal area. This is a very treatable condition and one not to miss (check serum erythrocyte sedimentation rate). Do not confuse spondylosis with spondylitis which is inflammation of the vertebrae (aetiology includes infections such as TB [Pott's disease] and inflammatory conditions such as ankylosing spondylitis).

A²

a. iv – Tangles of small rod-shaped granules in type I fibres are seen in nemaline myopathy. This congenital disorder is characterised by floppy infant syndrome and hypotonia at birth. However, the clinical picture can range from a mild, non-progressive disease to severe weakness ending in death from respiratory failure. A normal serum creatine kinase level is often seen.

b. viii – A ragged red appearance of muscle fibres on histology is characteristic of a mitochondrial myopathy. Mitochondrial myopathies demonstrate non-Mendelian inheritance. They are maternally transmitted DNA abnormalities in the mitochondria. For example, Kearns–Sayre syndrome is a mitochondrial myopathy.

c. iii – Denervation atrophy occurs due to muscle denervation. It involves type I and type II muscle fibres as well as target fibres, which have a central darker area resembling a bullseye. After re-innervation, fibre-type grouping, which is a group of type I fibres next to a group of type II fibres, can be seen.

d. i – A random variation in muscle fibre size and replacement of necrotic fibres by fibrofatty tissue are classic histological findings found in Duchenne muscular dystrophy. A lack of dystrophin, which anchors muscle fibres to the extracellular matrix, results in permanent damage. Muscle fibres that are irreversibly damaged are infiltrated by macrophages that replace them with collagen and adipose tissue.

e. vi – Continuous disuse of muscle, which is most commonly seen in bedridden older patients, results in atrophy. On histology, angular atrophy of type II muscle fibres is seen.[4]

A³

Correct answer is E – Creutzfeldt–Jakob disease

Creutzfeldt–Jakob disease is a prion disease that causes a rapidly progressive (weeks to months) dementia and early death. It can be acquired through ingestion of beef from cattle affected by mad cow disease. Prion diseases are caused by the conversion of a normal cellular protein termed *prion protein* to a beta-pleated form. The beta-pleated form resists degradation by proteases and its accumulation results in a spongiform encephalopathy. Multiple cysts with an absence of inflammatory cells on biopsy are characteristic.[5,6]

Parkinson's disease (answer A) results in a resting tremor, bradykinesia, rigidity and postural instability. Brain autopsy would reveal depigmentation of the substantia nigra.

HD (answer B) is an inherited condition. Basal ganglia degeneration is characteristic.

Pick's disease (answer C) causes fronto-temporal lobe dementia with atrophy. Pick bodies, which are intracellular and contain aggregated tau protein, are characteristic.

Alzheimer's dementia (answer D) is the most common cause of gradually progressing dementia. Beta-amyloid plaques and neurofibrillary tangles are characteristic.

References

1. Kumar P, Clark ML, editors. *Kumar & Clark's Clinical Medicine*. 7th ed. Edinburgh: Saunders Elsevier; 2009.
2. Goljan EF. *Rapid Review Pathology*. 3rd ed. Philadelphia, PA: Mosby/Elsevier; 2010.
3. Fitzgerald MJT, Gruener G, Mtui E. *Clinical Neuroanatomy and Neuroscience*. 5th ed. Edinburgh: Elsevier Saunders; 2007.
4. Schneider AS, Szanto PA. Musculoskeletal system. *Pathology*. 4th ed. Philadelphia, PA: Wolters Kluwer Health/Lippincott Williams & Wilkins; 2009. pp. 343–58.
5. Sikorska B, Knight R, Ironside JW, *et al*. Creutzfeldt–Jakob disease. *Adv Exp Med Biol*. 2012; **724**: 76–90.
6. Dastur DK, Manghani DK, Singhal BS. Histopathology and fine structure of the brain in six cases of Creutzfeldt–Jakob disease from western India. *J Neurol Sci*. 1992; **108**(2): 154–67.

10

Motor neurone disease

Q1 With regard to ALS, which of the following statements are true and which are false?

   a. ALS affects more men than women.

   b. The definitive diagnosis of ALS requires the demonstration of upper and lower motor neurone degeneration in at least four areas.

   c. It is inherited primarily in an autosomal recessive manner.

   d. ALS patients can develop fronto-temporal dementia.

   e. It is the reticulospinal tracts that are affected the most in ALS.

Q2 Regarding the treatment of MND, which of the following statements are true and which are false?

   a. Drug therapy targeting the release of the GABA neurotransmitter is the mainstay of treatment of MND.

   b. Non-invasive ventilation (NIV) is recommended in MND patients with a forced vital capacity (FVC) of <50%.

   c. Suxamethonium is an excellent drug that can be used to help reduce spasticity of the affected muscles.

   d. Pain experienced by patients with MND is most responsive to non-opioid analgesics.

Q3 The median survival for primary lateral sclerosis (PLS) is:
   a. <1 year
   b. 2–3 years
   c. 3–5 years
   d. 10–15 years
   e. 20+ years

Q4 A 37-year-old man visits his GP because of increasing difficulty in walking. There are fasciculations in all four limbs and increased tone in the legs. There is no sensory deficit. A presumptive diagnosis of ALS is made. If this diagnosis is correct, which of the following pharmacological treatments has been proven to lengthen survival rates in these patients?
   a. Donepezil
   b. Memantine
   c. Risperidone
   d. Riluzole
   e. Selegiline

Answers

A¹

a. TRUE – Studies have consistently shown this to be the case. Men are affected approximately 1.5 times more than women but this can vary with age.[1]

b. FALSE – According to the revised El Escorial Criteria, a definite diagnosis would require demonstration of degeneration of both upper and lower motor neurones in three areas with disease progression over time in these areas or to other areas. The diagnosis would also require absence of electrophysiological and neuroimaging evidence for other disease processes that might explain the upper and lower motor neurone signs.

c. FALSE – Familial ALS accounts for about 10% of cases (the rest being sporadic) and is *primarily* inherited in an autosomal dominant manner (at least 10 genes have been identified with SOD1 [superoxide dismutase 1] gene mutations accounting for 20% of all FALS). Four rare gene mutations have been implicated in autosomal recessive inheritance of FALS, and ALS15 (*UBQLN2*) is a rare gene encoding Ubiquilin-2 which has an X-linked mode of inheritance in FALS.[1]

d. TRUE – Approximately 30% develop mild to moderate cognitive defects but then 5% go on to develop overt fronto-temporal dementia.

e. FALSE – ALS is a multi-system disease affecting the motor pathways (descending tracts) but it is the corticospinal pathway that is primarily affected.[2]

A²

a. FALSE – Reducing the excess levels of glutamate, which is an excitatory neurotransmitter, may help to prevent the effect of excito-toxicity on motor neurones.

b. TRUE – National Institute for Health and Care Excellence guidelines recommend NIV for any MND patient with a FVC of <50% or a FVC of <80% plus one other symptom or sign of respiratory impairment including breathlessness, orthopnoea, increased respiratory rate and shallow breathing. For the full list of symptoms and signs *see* http://publications.nice.org.uk/motor-neurone-disease-cg105/guidance.[3]

c. FALSE – Suxamethonium is never used as a muscle relaxant except for under general anaesthesia. Botulinum toxin is often used to help combat the spasticity of muscles in MND patients.

d. FALSE – Pain can often be quite severe as a result of prolonged pulling on muscles, due to the spasticity that is a result of upper motor neurone degeneration, hence opioid analgesics can significantly improve the pain.

A[3]

Correct answer is E – 20+ years

PLS is a type of MND similar to ALS (Lou Gehrig's disease). The difference between the two types is that PLS is very slow progressing and only affects the upper motor neurones (ALS can affect upper and lower motor neurones). PLS leads to muscle hypertonia rather than atrophy. Occasionally, PLS may progress and convert to ALS.

A[4]

Correct answer is D – Riluzole

Patients with ALS display both upper and lower motor neurone signs. The patient in the scenario exhibits fasciculations, which is a lower motor neurone sign, and increased tone, which is an upper motor neurone sign. Another distinguishing feature of this disease process is the absence of sensory deficits.[4] Riluzole has been proven to effectively lengthen survival rates by 2–3 months (by slowing down disease progression) when used for 18 months.[5] It is a neuroprotective drug that inhibits the release of glutamate and blocks the effects of it on N-methyl-D-aspartate (NMDA) receptors, thereby preventing excitotoxicity-mediated damage to neurones.[6]

Donepezil (answer A) is used in Alzheimer's dementia. It is an acetylcholinesterase inhibitor.

Memantine (answer B) is also used in Alzheimer's dementia. It is an NMDA receptor antagonist and helps prevent excito-toxicity mediated by Ca^{2+}.

Risperidone (answer C) is an atypical antipsychotic drug often used in schizophrenia and bipolar disorders.

Selegiline (answer E) selectively inhibits monoamine oxidase B. It is commonly used as an adjunctive agent to l-dopa to treat Parkinson's disease.

References

1. Kinsley L, Siddique T. *Amyotrophic Lateral Sclerosis Overview.* 2001 Mar 23 [Updated 2012 May 31]. In: Pagon RA, Adam MP, Bird TD, *et al.*, editors. GeneReviews™ [Internet]. Seattle, WA: University of Washington, Seattle; 1993–2013. Available from: www.ncbi.nlm.nih.gov/books/NBK1450/ (accessed 20 August 2013).
2. Wijesekera LC, Leigh PN. Amyotrophic lateral sclerosis. *Orphanet J Rare Dis.* 2009; **4**: 3.
3. National Institute for Health and Care Excellence (NICE). Motor Neurone Disease: the use of non-invasive ventilation in the management of motor neurone disease; NICE guideline 105. London: NICE; 2010. http://publications.nice.org.uk/motor-neurone-disease-cg105 (accessed 10 January 2013).
4. Frosch MP, Anthony DC, De Girolami U. The central nervous system. In: Kumar V, Abbas AK, Fausto N, *et al. Robbins and Cotran Pathologic Basis of Disease, Professional Edition.* 8th ed. Philadelphia, PA: Saunders Elsevier; 2010.
5. Miller RG, Mitchell JD, Lyon M, *et al.* Riluzole for amyotrophic lateral sclerosis (ALS)/motor neuron disease (MND). *Cochrane Database Syst Rev.* 2007; 1: CD001447.
6. Rang HP, Dale MM, Ritter JM, *et al.* Neurodegenerative diseases. *Rang and Dale's Pharmacology.* 6th ed. New York, NY: Churchill Livingstone; 2007. p. 512.

11

Movement disorders

Q¹

    i. Stroke

   ii. Antalgic gait

  iii. Foot drop

  iv. Normal

   v. Charcot–Marie–Tooth disease

  vi. Cerebellar syndrome

 vii. Diabetes

viii. Spinal cord lesion

  ix. Parkinson's disease

Select from this list the most suitable diagnosis for the following gait disturbances.

a. An 11-year-old girl presented with clumsiness. On examination, she had a wide-based unsteady gait and a marked intention tremor.

b. A 65-year-old gentleman presented to the GP with monotonous speech, a resting tremor and a shuffling gait.

c. A 55-year-old lady presents to the GP with long-standing pain in her right knee. On examination, her gait seems extremely painful.

d. A 35-year-old presents with high-arched feet and a high-stepping gait. On further examination, there are 'inverted champagne bottle'-shaped legs.

Q2

i. Angelman syndrome

ii. Parkinson's disease

iii. Tardive dyskinesia

iv. Normal pressure hydrocephalus

v. Wernicke's encephalopathy

vi. HD

vii. Sydenham's chorea

viii. West syndrome

ix. GBS

Select from this list the answers to the following questions; the answers may be used once, more than once or not at all. What is the most accurate diagnosis in each patient?

a. A 49-year-old alcoholic is brought to the A&E department when his wife notices him having problems with his memory and difficulty walking and balancing. On examination, you note an ataxic gait and problems on downward and outward movement of the right eye. While you are speaking to him, the wife keeps correcting his story.

b. A 30-year-old man presents with an ascending weakness in his legs over the course of a few days. When you are taking his history you find out that he had gastroenteritis a couple of weeks ago. On examination you note hyporeflexia in his Achilles tendons bilaterally.

c. A 27-year-old man brings his 52-year-old father to the GP because of progressive rhythmic, uncontrollable twitching and dance-like movements in his extremities. The son reports his father's personality has changed over the years and he is having great difficulty with his memory. His grandfather also had very similar symptoms.

d. A normally healthy 7-month-old boy is brought to the A&E department by his parents. His parents were making a home video when they managed to catch him having a seizure; you see the child has been symmetrically jerking his head, arms and legs for around 1 minute. The boy appears to have had a post-ictal phase. He has met his developmental milestones so far.

e. A 40-year-old schizophrenic patient is brought to the A&E department by her sister, because she made tic-like movements with her lips and tongue. She was diagnosed with schizophrenia 10 months ago and has been managing it with medication, achieving a good degree of control over her symptoms.

Q3 A 60-year-old female presented with a 3-month history of progress-ive unsteadiness. She has a medical history of hypertension and right total mastectomy. Examination revealed marked difficulty with tandem walking, although sensation (including temperature and vibration) was normal and power was 4+/5 in both legs. What is the most likely diagnosis?

a. Stroke

b. MS

c. Vitamin B_{12} deficiency

d. Friedreich's ataxia

e. Paraneoplastic cerebellar degeneration

Q4 A 15-year-old male presents with a 3-year history of progressive ataxia and dysarthria. His medical history includes diabetes mellitus. What is the most likely diagnosis?

a. Friedreich's ataxia

b. Ataxia telangiectasia

c. MS

d. Sarcoidosis

e. Amyloidosis

Answers

A¹

a. vi – Cerebellar syndrome. Cerebellar symptoms can be remembered by the mnemonic 'DANISH':
    - **D**ysdiadochokinesis
    - **A**taxia
    - **N**ystagmus
    - **I**ntention tremor
    - **S**canning dysarthria
    - Hypotonia/positive **H**eel shin test

b. ix – Parkinson's disease. Characteristic features of Parkinson's disease are rigidity, bradykinesia, resting 'pill-rolling' tremor, mask-like appearance of the face, anosmia, micrographia and shuffling gait.

c. ii – Antalgic gait.

d. v – Charcot–Marie–Tooth disease. Charcot–Marie–Tooth disease is also known as hereditary motor and sensory neuropathy. It has a prevalence of 1 in 2500, making it one of the commonest inherited neurological diseases (usually autosomal dominant, although X-linked and recessive variants do exist). The usual symptoms include a progressive distal weakness of muscles and atrophy (hence the description 'inverted champagne bottles'), high-arched foot deformities, distal sensory loss and hyporeflexia.[1]

A²

a. v – The classic triad of ophthalmoplegia (paralysis of one or more eye muscles), ataxia and confusion is highly suggestive of Wernicke's encephalopathy. The patient is also starting to show signs of progression to Korsakoff's syndrome, which consists of memory lapses, confusion and confabulation. The ophthalmoplegia should distinguish this diagnosis from that of Parkinson's disease.[2]

b. ix – Also known as acute inflammatory demyelinating polyradiculopathy (AIDP). GBS is characterised by ascending muscle weakness commencing in the lower limbs. GBS is also associated with paraesthesia, hyporeflexia, cranial nerve deficits and may progress to respiratory muscle paralysis (cause of mortality). GBS has a prevalence of approximately 1 to 4 per 100 000 and has been associated with gastrointestinal infections with *Campylobacter jejuni*, upper respiratory tract infections and influenza vaccination (onset usually 1–3 weeks post infection).[3] Miller Fisher syndrome is very similar to GBS (a rare variant) except clinically there is a descending paralysis.

c. vi – HD is characterised by cognitive impairment (mainly forgetfulness and slowness of thought), motor disturbance of the face, arms, trunks, or legs (primarily chorea, although rigidity, bradykinesia and dystonia may be seen in late HD) and psychiatric disorders (commonly depression, anxiety, OCD and psychosis). It has an autosomal dominant pattern of genetic inheritance. HD is due to a mutation on chromosome 4 resulting in a repeat in the 'CAG' trinucleotide. Sydenham's chorea is associated with rheumatic fever. Tardive dyskinesia and Wilson's disease should also be included in the differential.[4]

d. viii – This is also known as infantile spasms. It is a rare form of generalised epilepsy in infants, affecting males more than females. It usually presents between 3 and 12 months of age, peaking at 5 months of age. These infants will stop psychomotor development at the age of the seizure onset, making the prognosis very poor and the disease very serious. A characteristic EEG finding is that of hypsarrhythmia (high amplitude and irregular waves and spikes in a background of chaotic and disorganised activity). Seizures are bilaterally symmetric flexion/extension movements of the arms, legs and trunk (hence these seizures are sometimes known as 'salaam' spasms or 'jack knife' convulsions). Individual spasms last only a few seconds, although they can occur in clusters lasting minutes.[5]

e. iii – Tardive dyskinesia is an extra-pyramidal symptom of typical antipsychotics. It manifests as stereotypical oral, buccal, lingual or choreiform movements. The other movement abnormalities associated with antipsychotic agents include *acute dystonia* (sustained muscular spasms – earliest sign), *akathisia* (extreme restlessness) and *akinesia* (inability to initiate movement).[6]

A³

Correct answer is E – Paraneoplastic cerebellar degeneration

Stroke is an incorrect answer as it is a sudden neurological deficit. MS is unlikely, as it usually presents at a younger age and symptoms would include muscle weakness. Vitamin B_{12} deficiency is also incorrect, since vibration sense is completely normal in this patient. Vitamin B_{12} deficiency can cause subacute combined degeneration of the cord; this affects the dorsal columns that carry proprioception and vibration. Friedreich's ataxia affects the young.

This patient has a history of mastectomy that is suggestive of previous breast cancer, and inability to tandem walk is a typical cerebellar sign (ataxia) (also dysdiadochokinesis, nystagmus, intention tremor, dysarthria and hypotonia). Therefore, paraneoplastic cerebellar degeneration is the most likely cause of the patient's symptoms. Paraneoplastic cerebellar degeneration is an autoimmune disease where antibodies are directed against Purkinje cells in the cerebellum. It is often associated with lung, breast and ovarian cancers and Hodgkin's lymphoma.[7]

A⁴

Correct answer is A – Friedreich's ataxia

This is an inherited autosomal recessive condition affecting patients commonly around 8–16 years of age. It is a trinucleotide repeat disorder of 'GAA' found in the frataxin gene. Patients commonly present with cerebellar signs. They can also have foot deformities (high-arched feet or pes cavus), diabetes mellitus and hypertrophic cardiomyopathy (a usual cause of death in these patients).[8]

References

1. Li J. Inherited neuropathies. *Semin Neurol.* 2012; **32**(3): 204–14.
2. Goljan EF. *Rapid Review Pathology.* 3rd ed. Philadelphia, PA: Mosby/Elsevier; 2010.
3. Fitzgerald MJT, Gruener G, Mtui E. *Clinical Neuroanatomy and Neuroscience.* 5th ed. Edinburgh: Elsevier Saunders, 2007.
4. Kumar P, Clark ML, editors. *Kumar & Clark's Clinical Medicine.* 7th ed. Edinburgh: Saunders Elsevier; 2009.

5. Swann JW, Moshe SL. On the Basic Mechanisms of Infantile Spasms. In: Noebels JL, Avoli M, Rogawski MA, *et al.*, editors. *Jasper's Basic Mechanisms of the Epilepsies* [Internet]. 4th ed. Bethesda, MD: National Center for Biotechnology Information (US); 2012. Available from: www.ncbi.nlm.nih.gov/books/NBK98133/.

6. Rang HP, Dale MM, Ritter JM, *et al. Rang and Dale's Pharmacology.* 6th ed. Edinburgh: Churchill Livingstone; 2007.

7. Ogita S, Llaguna OH, Feldman SM, *et al.* Paraneoplastic cerebellar degeneration with anti-Yo antibody in a patient with HER2/neu overexpressing breast cancer: a case report with a current literature review. *Breast J.* 2008; **14**(4): 382–4.

8. Haslett C, Chilvers ER, Boon N, editors. *Davidson's Principles and Practice of Medicine.* 19th ed. Edinburgh: Elsevier Science; 2002.

12

Neuroanatomy

Q¹

 i. Anterior radicular artery
 ii. Fasciculus gracilis
 iii. Fasciculus cuneatus
 iv. Corticospinal tract
 v. Ventral root
 vi. Dorsal root ganglion
 vii. Dorsal horn
 viii. Sympathetic chain
 ix. Anterior spinal artery
 x. Posterior spinal artery
 xi. Segmental medullary artery
 xii. Spinocerebellar tract

Choose the most appropriate answer from the list for each statement:

a. First-order neurones carrying vibration and proprioception sensations from the lower limb ascend in this area.

b. The soma of a neurone originating from a Meissner's corpuscle lies here.

c. This enables neurones from the thoracic region to enter the cranium and supply the dilator pupillae of the eye, causing mydriasis.

d. This artery supplies neurones in the spinal cord of the ventral corticospinal tract.

e. This artery supplies neurones carrying sensations of discriminative (fine) touch in the spinal cord.

Q2 Which of the following statements concerning the vascular anatomy of the head and neck are true and which are false?

   a. The innominate artery gives rise to the right subclavian and right common carotid arteries.

   b. The external carotid initially courses antero-laterally before curving posteriorly behind the mandible.

   c. Amaurosis fugax is caused by the occlusion of the occipital artery, a branch of the external carotid artery.

   d. Lacunar infarcts account for more than 20% of all strokes.

   e. A complete circle of Willis is present in more than 50% of patients.

Q3 Which of the following statements regarding the brachial plexus are true and which are false?

   a. Spinal nerves C5–T1 give rise to the roots of the brachial plexus that lie anatomically between the scalenus medius and posterior neck muscles.

   b. The ventral roots of spinal nerves contain sensory axons that convey information such as proprioception, pain and temperature.

   c. In a patient presenting with weakness and wasting of the hand and sensory loss on the inner aspect of the forearm and hand, it is important to do a chest X-ray.

   d. Shoulder dystocia during birth is a common cause of Erb's palsy.

   e. Spinal nerves C5–C7 usually give rise to the musculocutaneous nerve, which provides sensorimotor innervation to the upper arm, elbow and lateral aspects of the forearm.

Q4 Which of the following pass through the cavernous sinus?
   a. Optic nerve
   b. Oculomotor nerve
   c. Facial nerve
   d. Mandibular branch of the trigeminal nerve
   e. External carotid artery

Q5 The diagram shown is of a horizontal section through the cerebral cortex. Label the structures marked a–e with the appropriate structures from the following list.

    i. Globus pallidus

    ii. Third ventricle

    iii. Thalamus

    iv. Putamen

    v. Caudate nucleus

    vi. Corpus callosum

    vii. Internal capsule

    viii. Lateral ventricle

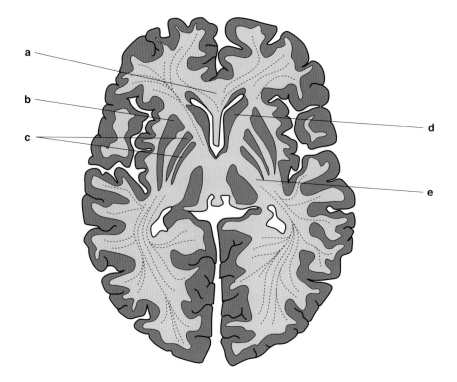

Answers

A¹

a. ii – Fasciculus gracilis. The dorsal columns consist of the fasciculus gracilis and fasciculus cuneatus, both consisting of neurones which convey proprioception, vibration, discriminative touch and pressure. Afferent sensory neurones entering the spinal cord below vertebral level T6 go on to form the fasciculus gracilis, and those entering above T6 form the fasciculus cuneatus.

b. vi – Dorsal root ganglion. Meissner's corpuscles are a type of mechanoreceptor arising from the skin; they convey sensations of light touch to the CNS. A pseudounipolar neurone would innervate the Meissner's corpuscle, whose soma (cell body) would lie in the dorsal root ganglion before it enters the spinal cord.

c. viii – Sympathetic chain. The sympathetic chain runs paravertebral in a bilateral fashion. Sympathetic nerves traverse the sympathetic chain from the thoracic region before entering the cervical ganglion and innervating the dilator pupillae of the eye.[1]

d. ix – Anterior spinal artery. The ventral corticospinal tract lies alongside the ventral part of the spinal cord and is closely related to the anterior spinal artery, which perfuses two-thirds of the spinal cord, including this tract.

e. x – Posterior spinal artery. Neurones carrying discriminative (fine) touch would ascend in the dorsal columns. The posterior spinal artery supplies the dorsal columns.[2]

A²

a. TRUE – The innominate artery, also known as the brachiocephalic artery, is the largest branch of the arch of the aorta. It divides into the right common carotid and right subclavian arteries. Usually the innominate artery does not have any branches, although occasionally the thyroidea ima artery (supplying the lower part of the thyroid) can arise from the innominate artery.

b. FALSE – It courses antero-medially then posteriorly and several branches of the external carotid are important collaterals if ever there is an occlusion of the internal carotid artery. It is possible to anatomically differentiate between the internal carotid and external carotid arteries by looking at the branches; the internal carotid usually has *no* branches in the neck. The branches of the external carotid are: superior thyroid, lingual, facial, maxillary, superficial temporal, posterior auricular, occipital and ascending pharyngeal.

c. FALSE – Amaurosis fugax is a transient curtain-like loss of vision and precedes central retinal artery occlusion (CRAO). The central retinal artery is a branch of the ophthalmic artery which arises from the internal carotid. Once CRAO occurs, it usually results in permanent monocular blindness. CRAO may be caused by an embolus (e.g. thrombotic), inflammatory diseases such as GCA and infection – for instance, toxoplasmosis. Certain drugs like cocaine can also cause vasoconstriction and lead to CRAO.[3]

d. TRUE – Lacunar infarcts involve the lenticulostriate arteries that supply the basal ganglia. The end arteries have very little or no collateral vascular supply. A major risk factor for intracerebral haemorrhage causing a thalamic bleed is hypertension (>70% of bleeds).[4]

e. FALSE – Only 25% of patients tend to have a complete circle of Willis.[5]

A³

a. FALSE – They lie between the scalenus anterior and medius muscles. Structures that pass between these muscles (the brachial plexus, subclavian artery and subclavian vein) may be compressed in what is known as thoracic outlet syndrome.

b. FALSE – Ventral roots contain alpha motor neurones that supply extrafusal striated muscle fibres, gamma motor neurones that supply intrafusal muscle spindles and also neurones with smaller diameters.[6]

c. TRUE – These symptoms suggest an apical tumour of the lung may have infiltrated the brachial plexus and this is known as Pancoast's syndrome.

d. TRUE – The dystocia may damage nerve roots C5 and C6. This usually leads to medial rotation of the arm as well as extension and pronation of the forearm (a position often described as 'waiter's tip').

e. TRUE – Lesions of this nerve usually result in weak flexion of the elbow, weak supination and sensory loss in the lateral aspects of the forearm. Lower motor neurone lesions also cause wasting and sometimes fasciculation.[7]

The following diagram is a schematic representation of the brachial plexus. It shows the roots C5–T1; note the contribution to the phrenic nerve that innervates the diaphragm ('C 3, 4, 5 keep the diaphragm alive'). The dorsal scapular nerve supplies the rhomboid muscles and levator scapulae muscle. The suprascapular nerve supplies supraspinatus and infraspinatus (two of the rotator cuff muscles; teres minor is supplied by the axillary nerve and subscapularis by the upper and lower subscapular nerves). The long thoracic nerve of Bell innervates the serratus anterior muscle and a lesion of this nerve results in winging of the scapula ('C 5, 6, 7 bells of heaven'). The axillary nerve supplies the deltoid muscles; this nerve is commonly injured in shoulder dislocations; always check the sensation over the 'regimental badge area' before attempting shoulder reduction to assess if damage has already occurred.

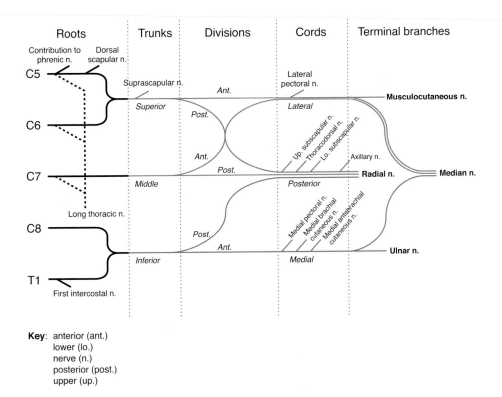

A⁴

Correct answer is B – Oculomotor nerve

The structures that pass through the cavernous sinus are the oculomotor nerve, trochlear nerve, ophthalmic and maxillary divisions of the trigeminal nerve, abducens nerve and the internal carotid artery.[8] The optic nerve passes superiorly and exteriorly to the cavernous sinus. The sinus itself receives a venous blood supply from the ophthalmic vein. Thus, the cavernous sinus is unique since an artery passes through a venous structure. A rupture of the internal carotid artery will cause an arterio-venous fistula (it is possible to hear an orbital bruit).[9] Patients can present with ophthalmoplegia, fixed dilated pupil, ptosis, proptosis, chemosis and facial pain. Treatment involves either neuroendovascular or neurosurgical approaches.

A⁵

a. vi – Corpus callosum
b. iv – Putamen
c. i – Globus pallidus
d. v – Caudate nucleus
e. vii – Internal capsule

References

1. Crossman AR, Neary D. *Neuroanatomy: an illustrated colour text.* 3rd ed. Edinburgh: Elsevier/Churchill Livingstone; 2005.
2. Thompson JC, Netter FH. *Netter's Concise Atlas of Orthopaedic Anatomy.* Philadelphia, PA: Saunders Elsevier; 2002.
3. Krishnaswamy A, Klein JP, Kapadia SR. Clinical cerebrovascular anatomy. *Catheter Cardiovasc Interv.* 2010; **75**(4): 530–9.
4. Kang CK, Park CA, Lee H, *et al.* Hypertension correlates with lenticulostriate arteries visualized by 7T magnetic resonance angiography. *Hypertension.* 2009; **54**(5): 1050–6.
5. Krabbe-Hartkamp MJ, van der Grond J, de Leeuw FE, *et al.* Circle of Willis: morphologic variation on three-dimensional time-of-flight MR angiograms. *Radiology.* 1998; **207**(1): 103–11.
6. Johnson EO, Vekris M, Demesticha T, *et al.* Neuroanatomy of the brachial plexus: normal and variant anatomy of its formation. *Surg Radiol Anat.* 2010; **32**(3): 291–7.

7. Knott L. *Musculocutaneous Nerve Lesion (C5–C6)*. Patient.co.uk; 2010. Available at: www.patient.co.uk/doctor/Musculocutaneous-Nerve-Lesion-%28C5-6%29.htm (accessed 10 January 2013).

8. Sharkawi E, Tumuluri K, Olver JM. Metastastic choriocarcinoma causing cavernous sinus syndrome. *Br J Ophthalmol*. 2006; **90**(5): 654–5.

9. Mitsuhashi T, Miyajima M, Saitoh R, *et al*. Spontaneous carotid-cavernous fistula in a patient with Ehlers-Danlos syndrome type IV: case report. *Neurol Med Chir (Tokyo)*. 2004; **44**(10): 548–53.

13

Neurodegeneration

Q¹

    i. HD

   ii. ALS

  iii. Parkinson's disease

  iv. Dementia with Lewy bodies

   v. Multiple system atrophy

  vi. Alzheimer's disease

 vii. Down's syndrome

viii. Prion disease

  ix. Pick's disease

   x. Progressive supranuclear palsy

  xi. Corticobasal degeneration

Match the following pathologies or clinical signs to the disease from the list shows that fits the description most accurately.

a. A disease characterised by the deposition of beta-amyloid plaques and neurofibrillary tangles.

b. A trinucleotide repeat expansion of 'CAG' often leads to this disease with choreoathetoid movements.

c. A resting tremor of 4–7 Hz, 'lead pipe' rigidity and bradykinesia are pathognomonic of this disease.

d. In this disease, degeneration within the brainstem leads to an inability of the patient to look vertically.

e. Adults with this hereditary disease almost invariably go on to develop Alzheimer's disease in later life.

2 With regard to Parkinson's disease, which of the following statements are true and which are false?

   a. Characteristic signs are a resting tremor, dysarthria and shuffling gait.

   b. Mutations in the SNCA and UCHL1 result in autosomal dominant inheritance of Parkinson's disease.

   c. Parkinson's disease is an alpha-synucleinopathy.

   d. Levodopa therapy improves dyskinesia in these patients.

   e. Supranuclear palsy is a non-degenerative cause of parkinsonism.

Q3 This diagram shows the direct and indirect pathways within the basal ganglia. The blue arrows represent glutamatergic neurotransmission (excitatory), the green arrows represent GABAergic neurotransmission (inhibitory) and the red arrows represent dopaminergic neurotransmission (excitatory for D_1 receptors and inhibitory for the D_2 receptors).

Match the parts of the basal ganglia labelled a–e with the following list of neuroanatomical structures.

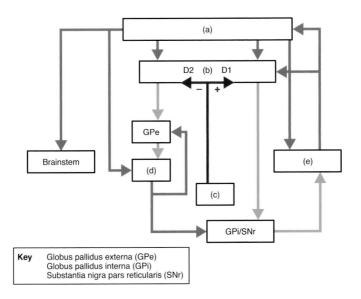

i. Subthalamic nucleus

ii. Corticospinal tract

iii. Substantia nigra pars compacta (SNc)

iv. Somatosensory cortex

v. Cerebral cortex

vi. Internal capsule

vii. Thalamus

viii. Claustrum

ix. Striatum

x. Nucleus basalis

4 Regarding Parkinson's disease, which of the following are true and which are false?

a. The motor symptoms are due to degeneration of dopaminergic neurones in the SNc.

b. Monoamine oxidase A inhibitors provide symptomatic benefit.

c. On histopathology, eosinophilic intracytoplasmic inclusions containing alpha-synuclein are seen.

d. Symptoms are often first seen when 30% of the dopaminergic neurones have degraded.

e. Rigidity, resting tremor and postural instability comprise the classic triad of cardinal signs.

5 A 73-year-old woman was brought to her GP by her husband, who explained that his wife was starting to become more forgetful. She was found to have a marked decline in cognitive ability and memory but an intact consciousness. No changes in sensation or movement were noted. Several years later, a post-mortem biopsy revealed beta-amyloid plaques and neurofibrillary tangles. Which part of the brain producing less neurotransmitter than usual is associated with this person's disease?

a. Locus coeruleus

b. Ventral tegmentum

c. Nucleus accumbens

d. Basal nucleus of Meynert

e. Raphe nucleus

Q6 A 72-year-old man presenting with forgetfulness, difficulty speaking and rigidity of movement undergoes a biopsy of a brain tissue sample. Intracellular and aggregated tau protein reveals Pick bodies and a diagnosis of Pick's disease (fronto-temporal dementia) is made. Which of the following types of hydrocephalus is most likely to be seen in this patient?

a. Normal pressure hydrocephalus

b. Hydrocephalus ex vacuo

c. Communicating hydrocephalus

d. Obstructive hydrocephalus

e. Non-communicating hydrocephalus

Q7 A 61-year-old woman has been recently diagnosed with Alzheimer's dementia. Some diagnostic features of dementia in general that can be used to differentiate it from delirium include the absence of psychotic symptoms and no change in the level of consciousness. What additional feature is a strong indicator of dementia that will help differentiate it from delirium?

a. A decrease in attention span

b. Disorganised thinking

c. Disturbance in the sleep–wake cycle

d. A gradual decrease in cognition

e. An abnormal EEG recording

Q8

   i. Frontal lobe atrophy
  ii. Diffuse cortical atrophy
 iii. Basal ganglia degeneration
  iv. Fronto-temporal atrophy
   v. Spongiform encephalopathy
  vi. Depigmentation of the substantia nigra
 vii. Lateral corticospinal tracts and ventral horn degeneration
viii. Atrophy of mammillary bodies, cerebellar vermis and pons
  ix. Degeneration of dorsal columns

Select a single best answer from the list provided that is most closely associated with each clinical scenario following.

a. A 34-year-old man presents to his GP with bilateral muscle weakness, increased spasticity and hyperreflexia of his legs. It is noted that there is unusual twitching of his right leg and muscular atrophy of both legs. No cognitive or sensory deficits are noted on nervous system examination.

b. A 41-year-old man is brought to his GP by his concerned wife. He is now aggressive and is not interested anymore in watching football matches, which he loved to do. His father also had a similar condition in his late 50s. On examination, choreiform movements are noted.

c. A 31-year-old woman presents to her GP because she has been extremely forgetful lately. Her husband explains that this started a couple of months ago and has become much worse since then. She has a wide-based gait and appears ataxic. Only a few years later, the woman dies from the disease causing her initial symptoms.

d. A 67-year-old man visits his GP with his wife. His GP notices that he seems to forget parts of their conversation they had just a couple of minutes ago. His wife reveals that once the police had to bring him home because he could not remember his way back from the local supermarket. The patient scores 14 on the Mini-Mental State Examination.

e. A 62-year-old woman is brought to the local practitioner by her daughter. The woman explains that her hands have become quite shaky recently and this is more prominent when she is sitting down to watch television. On examination, she is found to have a shuffling gait, increased tone in her arms and legs but scores 28 on the Mini-Mental State Examination.

Q9 Regarding Wilson's disease, which of the following are true and which are false?

a. It is autosomal dominant in nature.

b. It can be associated with osteoporosis.

c. The prevalence of the disease is approximately 1 in 30 000.

d. A liver transplant is the only way to prevent disease progression, even with an early diagnosis.

e. With treatment, functioning returns to before-disease levels.

Answers

A¹

a. vi – Alzheimer's disease

b. i – HD

c. iii – Parkinson's disease

d. x – Progressive supranuclear palsy

e. vii – Down's syndrome

A²

a. FALSE – The triad of signs that characterise Parkinson's disease are a resting tremor of 4–7 Hz with 'pill-rolling' movements, rigidity (often rigidity superimposed on tremor leads to a jerky resistance to passive movement known as 'cogwheeling') and bradykinesia with a difficulty in initiating movements.

b. TRUE – The SNCA (PARK1), UCHL1 (PARK5) and LRRK2 (PARK8) genes are linked to the autosomal dominant inheritance of Parkinson's disease, whilst PARK2, PARK7 and PINK1 (PARK6) are linked to autosomal recessive inheritance. However, the aforementioned genes account for the minority of Parkinson's cases whereas the majority are thought to arise from multiple gene effects and environmental risk factors.

c. TRUE – Neuronal eosinophilic inclusion bodies can be found in the SNc in Parkinson's patients. They can be elongated and branching within cellular processes (Lewy neuritis) or spherical within perikarya of neurones (Lewy bodies). They contain the misfolded protein alpha-synuclein. These inclusion bodies can be differentiated from other inclusion bodies – for instance, those found in synucleinopathies such as multiple system atrophy.[1]

d. FALSE – Dyskinesia in patients with Parkinson's disease is caused uniquely by levodopa therapy. It is not caused by other anti-Parkinson drugs. Almost 50% of patients on levodopa experience motor fluctuations and dyskinesias after 5 years. In the early stages of the disease, levodopa provides a long, smooth duration of clinical benefit by increasing the available levels of dopamine in the basal ganglia; this is because dopamine nerve terminals are able to store and release dopamine. However, as the disease progresses the duration of clinical benefit decreases and the concentration of levodopa in the basal ganglia becomes increasingly dependent on the plasma concentrations; this can lead to high levels of dopamine and hence abnormal involuntary movements known as dyskinesias. With regard to motor fluctuation, an 'on' period is when the patient experiences relief from symptoms as a result of pharmacological therapy, and an 'off' period is when the symptoms of Parkinson's disease return. Dyskinesias usually occur during the 'on' period.[2]

e. FALSE – It is a degenerative cause of parkinsonism and is known as a Parkinson plus disease since patients often suffer from a rapidly degenerating Parkinson-like disease with extra symptoms such as upward-gaze palsy. Non-degenerative causes of parkinsonism include drugs such as MPTP (methylphenyltetrahydropyridine), infections, vascular and metabolic causes.

A[3]

a. v – Cerebral cortex
b. ix – Striatum
c. iii – SNc
d. i – Subthalamic nucleus
e. vii – Thalamus

The motor cortex and the supplementary motor area predominantly project excitatory glutamatergic fibres to the spinal cord (lateral corticospinal tract), striatum and thalamus. The striatum consists of the caudate nucleus and the putamen, separated anatomically by the internal capsule. It comprises chiefly medium spiny neurones which are inherently inhibitory (GABAergic). The striatum projects inhibitory fibres to the globus pallidus interna (GPi) and substantia nigra pars reticularis (SNr). This pathway is known as the direct pathway since the GPi and SNr inhibit the thalamus (via the inhibitory ansa lenticularis projections) and hence if the striatum inhibits them, the thalamus is allowed to transmit excitatory output to the cerebral cortex and striatum (positive feedback loop).

The indirect pathway involves the striatum inhibiting the globus pallidus externa and hence un-inhibiting the subthalamic nucleus and therefore exciting the GPi and SNr, which then inhibit the thalamus. This is the exact opposite of what happens in the direct pathway. The SNc has dopaminergic projections to the striatum and the striatum has at least two types of dopamine receptors. D_1 receptors are excited by dopamine and result in activation of the direct pathway and hence lead to an increase in movement, whereas D_2 receptors are inhibited by dopamine and result in activation of the indirect pathway. Hence, dopaminergic loss in the putamen results in the hypokinetic state seen in Parkinson's disease, and loss of medium spiny neurones in the striatum leads to a hyperkinetic state seen in HD. Also, loss of dopamine in the caudate nucleus impairs executive functions and in limbic areas leads to depression.

A4

a. TRUE – Depletion of the dopaminergic neurones in the SNc gradually leads to denervation of the striatum and is the main cause of motor symptoms.[3]

b. FALSE – Dopamine is degraded by monoamine oxidase B. Inhibitors of this isoform, such as selegiline, are helpful in Parkinson's disease as they increase the availability of dopamine. Monoamine oxidase A preferentially metabolises serotonin and noradrenaline.[4]

c. TRUE – These inclusions are known as Lewy bodies; Parkinson's disease is associated with Lewy body formation.[3]

d. FALSE – Symptoms are more commonly produced when 50%–70% have degraded.[5]

e. FALSE – The classic triad comprises rigidity, resting tremor and bradykinesia.[5]

A5

Correct answer is D – Basal nucleus of Meynert

The basal nucleus of Meynert, found in the substantia innominata, is the major source of production of acetylcholine.[6] This is a classic case of Alzheimer's dementia, hinted at by the decline in cognitive function and the biopsy findings.[7] A decrease in acetylcholine due to atrophy of the basal nucleus of Meynert is strongly associated in patients with Alzheimer's dementia.[8]

The locus coeruleus (answer A) is the major site of production of noradrenaline. It can be associated with anxiety and depression, where there is an abnormally increased and decreased production, respectively.

The ventral tegmentum (answer B) produces dopamine, which is associated with a decrease in its production in Parkinson's disease.

The nucleus accumbens (answer C) produces GABA, which is associated with a decrease in its production in HD.

The raphe nucleus (answer E) produces serotonin, which is decreased in anxiety and depression.

A6

Correct answer is B – Hydrocephalus ex vacuo

Hydrocephalus ex vacuo is an increased appearance of CSF in atrophy of the brain. Dilation of the ventricles can also occur. This process is usually seen in Alzheimer's dementia, advanced HIV and Pick's disease. In contrast to other types of hydrocephalus, this type occurs due to a compensatory enlargement of the CSF spaces in response to parenchymal atrophy. It is not the result of increased CSF pressure, and ICP is normal in these patients.[7]

Normal pressure hydrocephalus (answer A) is a relatively common cause of reversible dementia. It results in the classic clinical triad of dementia, ataxia and urinary incontinence ('weird, wet and wobbly' is a common way of remembering the symptoms)

Communicating hydrocephalus (answer C) is caused by a decrease in CSF absorption by arachnoid villi, resulting in increased ICP, papilloedema and herniation.

Obstructive hydrocephalus (answer D) is caused by a structural blockage of CSF circulation within the ventricular system.

Non-communicating hydrocephalus (answer E) is a synonym for obstructive hydrocephalus.

A⁷

Correct answer is D – A gradual decrease in cognition

A gradual decrease in cognition over a long period of time is an additional strong indicator of dementia that will help differentiate it from delirium. Other features specific to dementia include a normal speech pattern and little diurnal variation in symptoms. Delirium usually presents secondary to an identifiable cause that has precipitated it. Specific features of delirium include the presence of psychotic symptoms (e.g. hallucinations), a fluctuating level of consciousness, an acute mode of onset and reversibility. The following table summarises the main differences between dementia and delirium.[9]

Dementia	Delirium
No psychotic symptoms	Psychotic symptoms
No change in the level of consciousness	Fluctuation in level of consciousness
A poor attention span in severe dementia	A poor but variable attention span (answer A)
Disorganised thinking only in late-stage dementia	Disorganised thinking (answer B)
Little to no disturbance in sleep–wake cycle	Disturbance in the sleep–wake cycle (answer C)
A gradual decrease in cognition	An abrupt decrease in cognition
A normal EEG recording	An abnormal EEG recording (answer E)

A⁸

a. vii – The history and findings are highly indicative of ALS. ALS can be caused by a defect in superoxide dismutase 1. Middle-aged patients usually present with upper and lower motor neurone signs with an absence of sensory or cognitive deficits. The typical presentation of this disease is due to degeneration of lateral corticospinal tracts and ventral horns in the spinal cord.[7] Riluzole, which decreases presynaptic glutamate release, has been proven to lengthen survival rates in these patients.[10]

b. iii – The history and findings most likely suggest that the patient is suffering from HD, which is a trinucleotide repeat disorder exhibiting an autosomal dominant inheritance pattern. Patients with this disease present at different ages, since it depends on when their predecessors experienced their first onset of symptoms. Basal ganglia degeneration and lower levels of GABA as well as acetylcholine in the brain are characteristic of this disease.[7]

c. v – A rapid-onset dementia with ataxia should always trigger the diagnosis of Creutzfeldt–Jakob disease. This prion disease is acquired and forms beta-pleated protein that is resistant to degradation. In turn, this process results in a characteristic spongiform encephalopathy. Patients with this disease have a very poor prognosis. Myoclonus can also be evident on examination.[11]

d. ii – This patient most likely has Alzheimer's dementia. The Mini-Mental State Examination suggests cognitive impairment. Patients with Alzheimer's dementia exhibit a gradual decline in cognitive ability and have widespread cortical atrophy on neuroimaging. The disease progress ranges from 8–10 years on average. Almost one quarter of cases are inherited (familial) but only 5% of these inherited cases occur before the age of 60.[7]

e. vi – Depigmentation of the substantia nigra is highly specific to Parkinson's disease. The typical presentation of a resting tremor, bradykinesia, rigidity and postural instability is characteristic. It is crucial to note that patients with Parkinson's disease *may* not have a decline in cognitive function but may be slow to express their thoughts.[9] The intact cognitive ability of this patient is indicated by the Mini-Mental State Examination score lying within the normal range.

A[9]

a. FALSE – Wilson's disease is autosomal *recessive*.

b. TRUE – Wilson's disease usually manifests with liver disease and clinical manifestation can vary from recurrent jaundice and self-limiting hepatitis to fulminant liver failure. Neurological disorders secondary to Wilson's can be classified as movement disorders (e.g. tremor and incoordination), or spastic dystonia disorders. Psychiatric manifestations of Wilson's are variable and include depression, compulsive behaviours, anxiety, aggression and disinhibition. Other clinical features that can also occur include osteoporosis in about 10% of cases, renal involvement, arthritis, pancreatitis and cardiomyopathy.[12]

c. TRUE – The prevalence of the disease is roughly 1 in 30 000, with most patients presenting within the ages of 5 and 40.

d. FALSE – Penicillamine can be used to chelate the copper so it can be excreted through the kidneys. However, it has a high rate of adverse effects and thus zinc or trientine (or a combination) can be used instead.

e. FALSE – Without treatment, the disease is usually fatal before 40 years of age. Only a limited amount of neurological function can be regained with early treatment but disease progression can be controlled, so further neurological or hepatic impairment can be prevented.

Some of the key features of Wilson's disease can be remembered by the following mnemonic:[13]

Worldwide prevalence 1 in 30 000 'Wing-beating' tremors
Inborn error of copper metabolism
Liver cirrhosis, low caeruloplasmin
Smile fixed (mask-like appearance) and slurring of speech (dysarthria)
Other: hepatitis, hepatomegaly, haemolysis
Neurological: ataxia, bradykinesia, chorea, dystonia, depression
D-penicillamine for treatment
Improper copper excretion
Spasticity and schizophrenia
Eyes: Kayser–Fleischer rings
Autosomal recessive
Serum copper decreased
Elevated urinary copper

References

1. Braak H, Del Tredici K, Bratzke H, *et al.* Staging of the intracerebral inclusion body pathology associated with idiopathic Parkinson's disease (preclinical and clinical stages). *J Neurol.* 2002; **249**(Suppl. 3): III/1–5.
2. Tarsy D. *Motor Fluctuations and Dyskinesia in Parkinson Disease.* Waltham, MA: UpToDate; 2010. Available at: www.uptodate.com/contents/motor-fluctuations-and-dyskinesia-in-parkinson-disease (accessed on 10 January 2013).
3. Kumar P, Clark M, editors. *Kumar and Clark's Clinical Medicine.* 7th ed. Edinburgh: Saunders Elsevier; 2009.

4. Golan DE, Tashjian AH, Armstrong EJ, *et al. Principles of Pharmacology: the patho-physiologic basis of drug therapy*. 3rd ed. Philadelphia, PA: Lippincott Williams & Wilkins; 2012.

5. Fauci A, Braunwald E, Kasper D, *et al.*, editors. *Harrison's Principles of Internal Medicine*. 17th ed. New York, NY: McGraw-Hill; 2008.

6. Schliebs R, Arendt T. The cholinergic system in aging and neuronal degeneration. *Behav Brain Res*. 2011; **221**(2): 555–63.

7. Frosch MP, Anthony DC, De Girolami U. The central nervous system. In: Kumar V, Abbas AK, Fausto N, *et al. Robbins and Cotran Pathologic Basis of Disease, Professional Edition*. 8th ed. Philadelphia, PA: Saunders Elsevier; 2010.

8. Grothe M, Zaborszky L, Atienza M, *et al.* Reduction of basal forebrain cholinergic system parallels cognitive impairment in patients at high risk of developing Alzheimer's disease. *Cereb Cortex*. 2010; **20**(7): 1685–95.

9. Bowker LK, Price JD, Smith SC. Psychiatry. *Oxford Handbook of Geriatric Medicine*. Oxford: Oxford University Press; 2006. pp. 219–76.

10. Miller RG, Mitchell JD, Lyon M, *et al.* Riluzole for amyotrophic lateral sclerosis (ALS)/motor neuron disease (MND). *Cochrane Database Syst Rev*. 2007; 1: CD001447.

11. Sikorska B, Knight R, Ironside JW, *et al.* Creutzfeldt–Jakob disease. *Adv Exp Med Biol*. 2012; **724**: 76–90.

12. Weiss KH. *Wilson Disease*. GeneReviews™. Seattle (WA): University of Washington, Seattle; 1993–2013. Available at: www.ncbi.nlm.nih.gov/books/NBK1512/ (accessed 10 January 2013).

13. Parmer HB. *Mnemonics in Internal Medicine and Pediatrics*. 1st ed. New Delhi: B. Jain Publishers; 2002.

14

Neuroimaging

Q1   A 69-year-old woman has been referred to the neurology clinic regarding a pain in the back of her neck and a palpable mass in the cervical region. She complains of tingling in her upper limbs. On examination, her upper limb power is recorded as grade 4 on the left and grade 5 on the right side. Upper limb reflexes are significantly diminished bilaterally. In order to identify potential intra-foraminal and epidural extension of the mass, which neuro-radiological modality is most appropriate?

a. Plain CT

b. X-ray

c. Ultrasound

d. MRI

e. CT myelography

2 Choose the most appropriate first-line investigation for each of the following cases.

   i. CT

   ii. T_1/T_2-weighted MRI

  iii. X-ray

  iv. Gadolinium-enhanced MRI

   v. Ultrasound

  vi. Diffusion-weighted MRI

 vii. Functional MRI

viii. MRI

  ix. Discogram

   x. Bone scintigraphy

a. A 1-week-old neonate is highly suspected of having a lipomyelomeningocele and the diagnosis needs evaluating.

b. A 53-year-old man presented with sudden severe lower back pain after lifting a heavy box at work. He has experienced symptoms of sciatica and has a prominent foot drop on gait examination. He has a medical history of hepatorenal syndrome. A spinal disc prolapse is highly probable.

c. A research scientist wishes to study the spinal activity of patients during motor tasks.

d. A researcher in neuroscience wishes to study the benefits on axonal integrity of a new drug for MS.

e. A 28-year-old man suffered blunt trauma to the side of his head and has a progressively deteriorating conscious level, severe headache and unilateral mydriasis. The Foundation Year 2 doctor suspects an extradural haemorrhage.

Q3 A 52-year-old female presents to the A&E department with a history of sudden-onset occipital headache and vomiting prior to collapsing at work. She is opening her eyes to pain, has incomprehensible speech and is withdrawing from pain. She has a medical history of autosomal dominant polycystic kidney disease. On examination, her pulse is 110 bpm and regular, and blood pressure is 182/107 mmHg with a right-sided hemiplegia. A CT scan is requested.

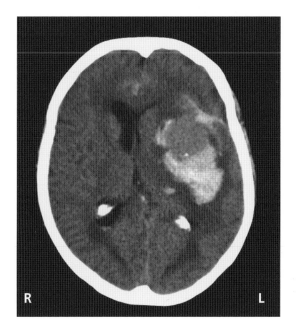

PART A

From this history and the CT scan, please select the most suitable diagnosis.

a. Subdural haemorrhage

b. SAH

c. Meningitis

d. Encephalitis

e. Cerebral venous sinus thrombosis

PART B

If the patient had a Glasgow Coma Scale score of 15 with no focal neuro-logical deficit and the CT scan was normal, which subsequent test would you perform to support this diagnosis?

a. Lumbar puncture

b. MRI with fluid-attenuated inversion recovery

c. Contrast CT

d. Carotid Doppler

e. Magnetic resonance angiogram

Q4 A 34-year-old rugby player received a head injury after being tackled by the opposing team. Initially he developed a headache and loss of consciousness prior to a slight recovery before a delayed decline in mental status. On examination, his pulse was 50 bpm, and his blood pressure was 142/92 mmHg with a Glasgow Coma Scale score of 13/15 and no focal neurological deficit. A CT scan was requested.

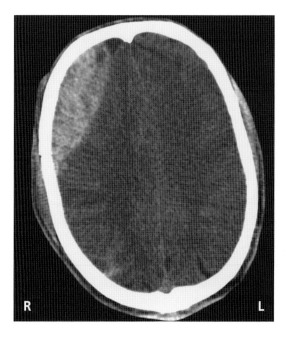

Please select the most suitable diagnosis.

a. Acute subdural haemorrhage

b. SAH

c. Chronic subdural haemorrhage

d. Extradural haemorrhage

e. Meningitis

Q5 A 79-year-old woman presents to the acute medical unit with a head-ache. Her family describes her as being very forgetful after having a fall a few weeks ago. On examination, there is no focal neurological deficit. A CT scan is requested.

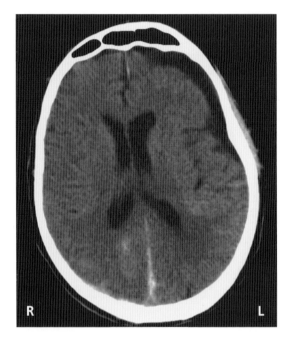

Please state the single most appropriate diagnosis.

a. Acute on CSDH

b. Extradural haematoma

c. SAH

d. Dementia

e. CSDH

Q6 A 25-year-old known intravenous drug user presents to the A&E
department with increasing confusion, headache and a fever. Initial
investigations are conducted, including a CT scan of the head.

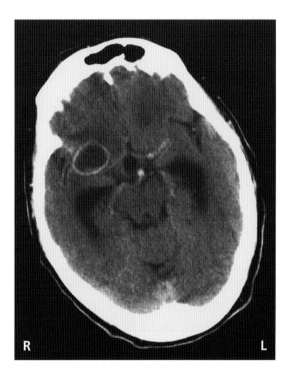

Please select the most suitable diagnosis.

a. Brain metastasis

b. Glioma

c. Intracranial abscess

d. Meningitis

e. Encephalitis

Q7 Which of the following statements regarding the T_2-weighted MRI scan shown here are true and which are false?

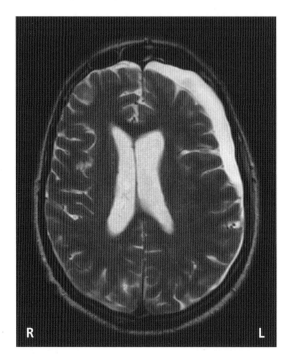

a. SAH
b. Left-sided subdural haematoma
c. Mass effect by the presence of a cerebral tumour
d. Middle meningeal artery tear
e. Effacement of the cortical sulci on the left hemisphere

Q8 A 64-year-old man presented having had a fall. He did not sustain any injuries to his head. History revealed the patient had been suffering from dementia. Examination showed no focal neurological deficit and fundoscopy was normal, although it was noted that he had gait disturbance. The patient also reported that for some time now he had been suffering with urinary incontinence. Based on the history and examination and the following T_2-weighted MRI scan, what is the most likely diagnosis?

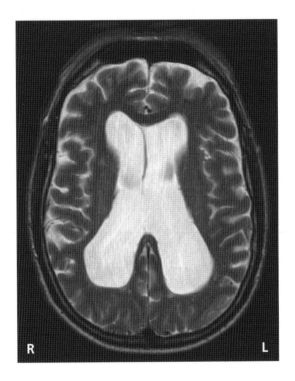

a. Parkinson's disease

b. Multi-infarct dementia

c. Middle cerebral artery stroke

d. Normal pressure hydrocephalous

e. Metastatic carcinoma

Q9 The following sagittal T$_2$-weighted MRI scan is from an 80-year-old man who had gait disturbances, a positive Rhomberg's test and in who nerve conduction studies had shown a mixed motor and sensory axonal-type polyneuropathy. The patient was known to have pernicious anaemia. What is the most likely diagnosis?

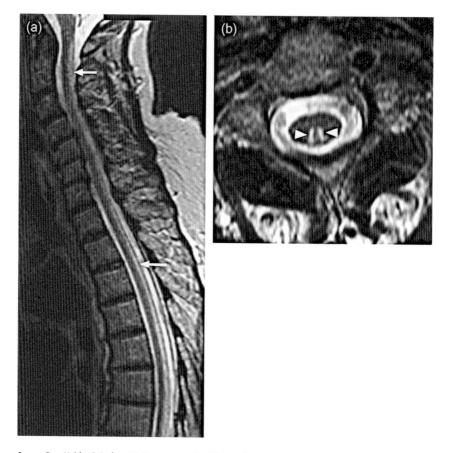

Source: Bou-Haider P, Peduto AJ, Karunaratne N. Differential diagnosis of T2 hyperintense spinal cord lesions: Part B. *Journal of Medical Imaging and Radiation Oncology.* 2009; **53**(2): 152–9. Reproduced with the kind permission of Wiley.

a. MS
b. Posterior spinal artery infarct
c. Subacute combined degeneration of the spinal cord
d. Transverse myelitis
e. Neurosarcoidosis

Q10 Match the image to the most likely diagnoses listed here.

    i. Metastatic tumour

    ii. Meningioma

    iii. Arachnoid cyst

    iv. GBM

    v. Pituitary tumour

    vi. Schwannoma

a.

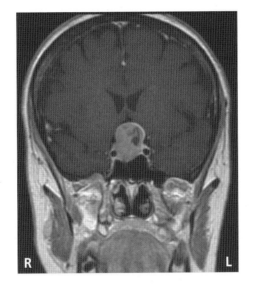

b.

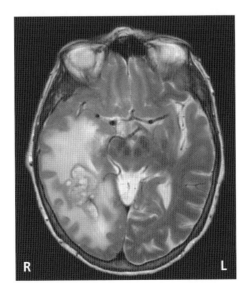

c.

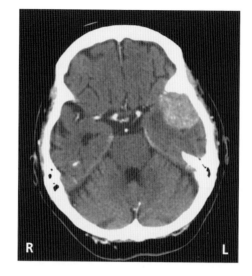

d.

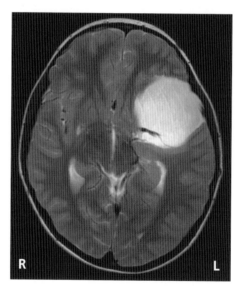

Answers

A¹

Correct answer is D – MRI

MRI is most appropriate since it does not involve ionising radiation, and provides detailed imaging enabling a clinician to accurately view intra-foraminal and epidural extension of a mass. A CT myelogram would also demonstrate this detail; however, this would mean the patient would unnecessarily have a dye injected into their dural sac and be exposed to radiation. CT myelograms are performed when patients have contraindications for MRI scans.

A²

a. v – Ultrasound. Due to the young age of the child and the lipomatous tissue being highly echogenic, an ultrasound would be the most appropriate scan to use in this situation.[1]

b. ii – T_1/T_2-weighted MRI. An MRI scan is the most appropriate method of choice here.[2] A gadolinium-enhanced scan is unnecessary and contraindicated because of the patient's hepatorenal syndrome.[3] The other options would be appropriate for more specific investigations.

c. vii – Functional MRI. A functional MRI scan would detect patterns of activity in the spinal cord in concordance with known physiology.[4] This would enable the researcher to view all activity within the spinal cord, whereas none of the other scans listed would display the activity in this way.

d. viii – Magnetic resonance spectroscopy. Magnetic resonance spectroscopy assesses the biochemical nature of tissues, which would provide a basis to study changes in axonal integrity.[5]

e. i – CT. A CT scan is the gold standard to accurately identify an extradural haemorrhage, which would usually display a biconvex haematoma.[2]

A³

PART A

Correct answer is B – SAH

The CT scan (in the question) shows a large left middle cerebral artery aneurysm with surrounding intraparenchymal and subarachnoid blood. There is also evidence of midline shift and compression of the left lateral ventricle. The three-dimensional reconstruction that is created following a CT angiogram shows the aneurysm on the left side.

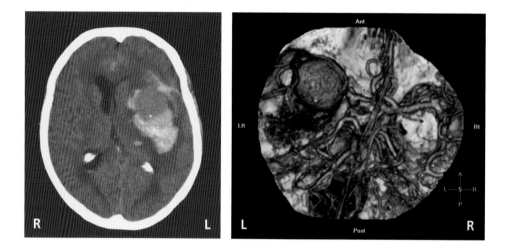

PART B

Correct answer is A – Lumbar puncture

If the CT scan was normal and SAH was suspected then it is imperative to perform a lumbar puncture, given that approximately 2% of SAHs are not seen on CT or MRI alone. A lumbar puncture is usually performed 12 hours after the onset of the headache. This delay is essential, because if there are red cells in the CSF, sufficient lysis will have taken place during that time for bilirubin and oxyhaemoglobin to have given the CSF a yellow tinge after centrifugation known as xanthochromia.[6] Xanthochromia can remain for up to 2 weeks after ictus (onset of SAH).

A⁴

Correct answer is D – Extradural haemorrhage

The CT scan shows an extradural haemorrhage with a hyperdense lenticular-shaped mass situated between the brain and the skull. In this case the patient experienced a typical lucid interval with loss of consciousness at the time of impact before experiencing an altered mental status. Also note that the extent of bleeding does not cross the suture lines. These patients need to be discussed urgently with the neurosurgical team, as decompensation and death can occur very quickly if untreated, especially in the moderate to large extradural haemorrhage.

A⁵

Correct answer is E – CSDH

There is a hypodense sickle-shaped extra-axial fluid collection with surrounding mass effect over the left cerebral hemisphere (representing old blood). There are three phases of a subdural haematoma.[7]

1. Hyperdense (1–3 days): fresh blood has higher attenuation on the CT scan (appears whiter) than the cerebral cortex. CSF fluid appears black (has low attenuation).
2. Isodense (3–21 days): the blood now has a very similar attenuation to the cerebral cortex and therefore it can be difficult to distinguish the bleed from the brain tissue. During this stage, in order to identify a subdural haematoma, indirect effects have to be examined: the CSF-filled sulci may not reach the skull, there may be mass effect (e.g. distortion of sulci or midline shift) and the cortex may appear thickened.
3. Hypodense (>21 days): the blood now starts to have an even lower attenuation than the brain tissue and after several days starts to appear more like the CSF fluid, which has a low attenuation as well.

A6

Correct answer is C – Intracranial abscess

The CT scan shows a ring enhancement on the right side of the brain. It is circular in nature with a highly attenuated ringed wall with low attenuation in its centre.[8] A developing intracranial abscess usually passes through three clinical stages.

1. Initial stage: malaise, fever, headache and primary source of the infection.
2. Latent stage: these symptoms resolve but there is a rise in ICP.
3. Space-occupying lesion.

In this case the abscess was caused due to infective endocarditis through intra-venous drug use, which is normally caused by a haematogenous *Staphylococcus aureus* or *Streptococcus viridans* infection.

A7

a. FALSE – SAHs are arterial bleeds that tend to follow the contours of the cerebral sulci. The patient classically complains of a 'thunderclap' headache. A CT scan is indicated acutely. Lumbar puncture can help confirm the diagnosis – look for xanthochromia.

b. TRUE – Subdural haematomas are usually venous haemorrhages and the MRI scan shows a crescent-shaped mass on the left hemisphere.

c. FALSE – Although there is a midline shift and mass effect, this is due to the presence of blood and not because of a tumour.

d. FALSE – Middle meningeal artery tears cause extradural haemorrhages and thus on an MRI scan there would be a biconvex mass, and, since this can sometimes look like a lens, they can be described as lentiform.

e. TRUE – The pressure as a result of the blood around the left cortical hemisphere compresses the brain and hence there is effacement of the sulci on the MRI scan.

A⁸

Correct answer is D – Normal pressure hydrocephalous

Normal pressure hydrocephalous is defined as a progressive disorder, without identifiable cause, that results in reported and observed gait ataxia, cognitive loss and/or urinary incontinence, accompanied by imaging evidence of ventriculomegaly. This is seen on the CT scan where the lateral ventricles appear significantly enlarged with respect to the size of the cranium. One way to remember the triad for normal pressure hydrocephalous is 'weird, wet and wobbly' – Hakim's triad of confusion, incontinence and ataxia.[9]

A⁹

Correct answer is C – Subacute combined degeneration of the spinal cord

Subacute combined degeneration of the spinal cord normally results from vitamin B_{12} (cobalamin) deficiency. The fact that this patient has pernicious anaemia is very important, since it is caused by a loss of gastric parietal cells, which are necessary for the production of intrinsic factor, without which vitamin B_{12} cannot be absorbed effectively.[10]

The mechanism of myelin damage is related to the reduced activity of the methylcobalamin esterase enzyme subsequently leading to an increase in methylmalonic acid, which is damaging to myelin.

The damage occurs predominantly in the dorsal columns of the spinal cord and thus a clinical feature of subacute combined degeneration of the cord is a positive Rhomberg's test due to impaired proprioception. The MRI scan shows high T_2 signal in the posterior aspect of the spinal cord spanning several segments. In MS, for example, the lesions are asymmetrical and usually 2–60 mm in length and oval shaped.[11]

A¹⁰

a. v – Pituitary tumour. Pituitary tumours are classified into microadenomas (<10 mm) and macroadenomas (>10 mm). Microadenomas are commonly asymptomatic as they are usually confined to the sella and have little potential for mass effect. However, they can be diagnosed when investigating hormonal imbalance in patients (e.g. excess production of prolactin). Macroadenomas can cause optic chiasm compression leading to bitemporal hemianopia. They can be locally invasive and intrude the cavernous sinus (usually prolactin secreting macroadenomas), although once this happens, complete surgical resection can become extremely difficult. A T_1/T_2-weighted MRI scan is the modality of choice. The adenoma appears isointense with the grey matter on this type of imaging. Trans-sphenoidal surgical resection is the mainstay of treatment. Differential diagnoses for pituitary macroadenomas include craniopharyngioma, metastasis, pituitary carcinoma and meningioma.

b. iv – GBM. It is the most common *primary* intracranial tumour. It enlarges rapidly and is often associated with neovascularity and necrosis. It is frequently localised in the frontal and temporal lobes. Patients with GBM commonly present with seizures or focal neurological deficits depending on the site of the tumour. An axial T_1/T_2-weighted MRI scan usually shows an infiltrating mass which contains a necrotic area in the middle. It usually crosses the corpus callosum too. Abscess and primary CNS lymphoma are the main differential diagnoses. Tumour de-bulking with chemo- or radiotherapy is the usual treatment.

c. ii – Meningioma. This is usually a benign slow-growing tumour that occasionally compresses adjacent structures. Less than 10% are symptomatic and symptoms are location dependent. A T_1/T_2-weighted MRI scan with contrast is the recommended modality of imaging. It commonly shows an intense homogeneously enhancing mass with a dural tail. The following side-by-side images are a comparison of the same meningioma as seen on a T_2-weighted MRI scan (left) and a normal CT scan of the head (right).

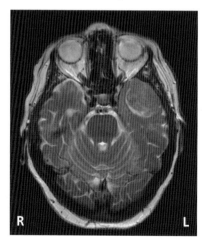 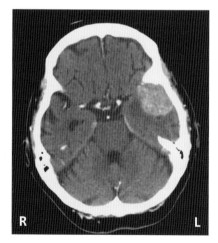

d. iii – Arachnoid cyst. It is an intra-arachnoid sac that is filled with CSF
without being connected to the ventricular system. It is the most
common congenital intracranial cystic abnormality. However, it makes
up around 1% of all intracranial masses. Fifty per cent of arachnoid
cysts are located in the middle cranial fossa. Epidermoid cyst is the
top differential diagnosis. They are often asymptomatic and found
incidentally. MRI with fluid-attenuated inversion recovery is the best
diagnostic imaging modality. It is usually left without treatment.[12] The
following side-by-side images are a comparison of the same arachnoid
cyst as seen on a T_2-weighted MRI scan (left) and a normal CT scan of
the head (right).

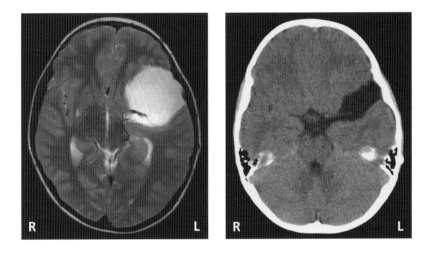

References

1. Blount JP, Elton S. Spinal lipomas. *Neurosurg Focus*. 2001; **10**(1): e3.
2. Longmore M, Wilkinson IB, Davidson EH, *et al*. *Oxford Handbook of Clinical Medicine*. 8th ed. New York, NY: Oxford University Press; 2010.
3. US Food and Drug Administration (FDA). *Questions and Answers on Gadolinium-Based Contrast Agents*. Silver Spring, MD: FDA; 2013. Available at: www.fda.gov/Drugs/DrugSafety/DrugSafetyNewsletter/ucm142889.htm (accessed 10 January 2013).
4. Kornelsen J, Stroman PW. fMRI of the lumbar spinal cord during a lower limb motor task. *Magn Reson Med*. 2004; **52**(2): 411–14.
5. De Stefano N, Narayanan S, Matthews PM, *et al*. Proton MR spectroscopy to assess axonal damage in multiple sclerosis and other white matter disorders. *J Neurovirol*. 2000; **6**(Suppl. 2): S121–9.

6. Van Gijn J, Rinkel GJ. Subarachnoid haemorrhage: diagnosis, causes and management. *Brain*. 2001; **124**(Pt. 2): 249–78.

7. Plaha P, Malhotra NR, Heuer GG, *et al*. Management of chronic subdural haematoma. *Adv Clin Neurosci Rehabil*. 2008; **8**(5): 12–15.

8. Shaw MD, Russell JA. Value of computed tomography in the diagnosis of intracranial abscess. *J Neurol Neurosurg Psychiatry*. 1977; **40**(3): 214–20.

9. Rosseau G. Normal pressure hydrocephalus. *Dis Mon*. 2011; **57**(10): 615–24.

10. Annibale B, Lahner E, Fave GD. Diagnosis and management of pernicious anemia. *Curr Gastroenterol Rep*. 2011; **13**(6): 518–24.

11. Bou-Haidar P, Peduto AJ, Karunaratne N. Differential diagnosis of T2 hyperintense spinal cord lesions: part B. *J Med Imaging Radiat Oncol*. 2009; **53**(2): 152–9.

12. Osborn AG, Salzman KL, Barkovich AJ, *et al*. *Diagnostic Imaging: brain*. 2nd ed. Salt Lake City, UT: Amirsys; 2010.

15

Peripheral neuropathy

Q1 In CTS, which of the following are true and which are false?

a. The radial nerve is compressed, leading to paraesthesia, numbness and weakness of the muscles of the hand.

b. It is more common in women early in their pregnancy.

c. Phalen's manoeuvre is used to help diagnose CTS clinically and is performed by extending the wrist and holding it in acute extension.

d. Tinel's sign is the reproduction of pain (or numbness and tingling) over the distribution of the compressed nerve by tapping over the flexor retinaculum.

e. There is weakness of the flexor pollicis brevis, opponens pollicis and abductor pollicis brevis.

Q2 A 23-year-old man presented with sensory loss in the medial half of the ring finger and small finger of the right hand. There was also weakness of the intrinsic muscles of the hand and weakness in the flexors of the ring and little finger. The abductor pollicis brevis was preserved. What is the most likely cause?

a. CTS

b. Musculocutaneous nerve lesion

c. T1 nerve root lesion

d. Distal radial nerve compression

e. Ulnar nerve entrapment

Q3 Match the following causes or types of peripheral neuropathy to the patient histories described.

   i. Diabetes

   ii. Charcot–Marie–Tooth disease

   iii. Hypothyroidism

   iv. Polyarteritis nodosa (PAN)

   v. Alcoholism

   vi. Chronic inflammatory demyelinating polyneuropathy

   vii. Vitamin B_{12} deficiency

   viii. GBS

   ix. Herpes zoster

   x. Lyme disease

a. A 56-year-old woman presents complaining of severe right lower limb pain. Physical examination is unremarkable except for a grouped vesicular lesion in a dermatomal distribution on the posterior aspect of her right leg. The patient subsequently developed right lower leg weakness 2 weeks later and began 'dragging' her foot while walking.

b. A 35-year-old man presents with generalised muscle aches of the upper and lower limbs. He has also been feeling weak and reports easily being fatigued. Physical examination reveals that the patient has a mottled purplish skin rash over his torso and has reduced sensation in the distal aspects of his lower limbs. His erythrocyte sedimentation rate and C-reactive protein are also raised.

c. A 47-year-old woman has paraesthesia and severe pain in her left hand. The pain is usually worse after she returns from work as an IT administrator. Recently, she has put on weight and experienced some hair loss. On examination, she has wasting of the thenar muscle group and Tinel's sign is positive. She is also bradycardic with a pulse of 49 bpm.

d. An 80-year-old man presents having had a fall. He reports that he awoke one morning and proceeded to make breakfast when his legs 'suddenly gave way' and he fell. A full neurological examination of the lower limbs shows the patient has absent ankle and knee reflexes and the plantars are unequivocal. Also, there is marked weakness in ankle plantarflexion and dorsiflexion and some weakness in knee flexion and extension. The next day, a repeat examination shows the weakness has affected his hip flexion and extension now.

e. A 25-year-old man presents with flu-like symptoms and a rash that has a characteristic 'bullseye' appearance. He is treated with doxycycline for 10 days. However, 4 weeks later his symptoms have persisted and now the patient is complaining of generalised muscle aches, palpitations and paraesthesia of his hands and feet. On examination, you notice the rash has not subsided and that the patient has 'patchy' sensory loss of the lower limbs.

Q4 Match the following answers to the appropriate clinical vignette. Each answer may be used more than once.

   i. Anti-voltage-gated calcium channel antibodies

   ii. MS

   iii. Low serum caeruloplasmin levels

   iv. Anti-nicotinic AChR-Ab

   v. Chronic inflammatory demyelinating polyneuropathy

   vi. GBS

   vii. Wet beri beri

   viii. PLS

   ix. Subacute combined degeneration of the spinal cord

   x. Dry beri beri

a. A 43-year-old alcoholic man is found to have symmetrical lower limb weakness and sensory loss. There is absence of the ankle jerk reflex on examination.

b. A 67-year-old lady with a recent diagnosis of small cell lung cancer is complaining of significant, progressive lower limb weakness. She also mentions having a dry mouth and feeling faint upon standing.

c. A 22-year-old man presents with an ascending motor paralysis of the legs that has got worse over the previous 2 days. He has recently recovered from gastroenteritis.

d. An older lady complains of tingling in her fingers and toes, long-standing lethargy and increasing shortness of breath. On examination, her tongue is very red and smooth and there is a sensory loss of vibration and proprioception over the distal limbs.

Answers

A¹

a. FALSE – There is median nerve compression.

b. FALSE – It is more common in late pregnancy when there is more fluid retention and there is a similar situation in patients with hypothyroidism who may then develop CTS.

c. FALSE – This manoeuvre is performed by holding the wrist in acute flexion and the development of numbness within 60 seconds is a positive sign.

d. TRUE

e. TRUE – There is usually wasting of the thenar eminence as well as sensory loss along the distribution of the median nerve.

A useful mnemonic for remembering the causes of CTS is 'MEDIAN TRAP':

Myxoedema, (o)**E**dema, **D**iabetes mellitus, **I**diopathic, **A**cromegaly, **N**eoplasm, **T**rauma, **R**heumatoid arthritis, **A**myloidosis and **P**regnancy

A²

Correct answer is E – Ulnar nerve entrapment

The ulnar nerve supplies the flexor carpi ulnaris and the ulnar half of the flexor digitorum profundus in the forearm. In the hand, it supplies the hypothenar muscles, which include the opponens digiti minimi, abductor digiti minimi and flexor digiti minimi, and also supplies the medial two lumbricals, dorsal interossei, palmar interossei and adductor pollicis.

A lesion of the ulnar nerve causes weakness of the flexors of the ring and little fingers. This causes hyperextension at the fourth and fifth metacarpophalyngeal joints. If the ulnar nerve lesion is closer to the hand (e.g. at Guyon's canal), the flexor digitorum profundus muscle (which originates in the forearm and is supplied in part by the ulnar nerve) can still contract leading to flexion of the fourth and fifth distal and proximal interphalangeal joints and hence a prominent claw hand. However, if the ulnar nerve lesion is more proximal (e.g. at the cubital tunnel at the elbow), the flexor digitorum profundus is denervated and hence flexion of the interphalyngeal joints does not occur and hence the ring and little fingers are held fixed in extension (less claw hand).

This is highly unusual as more proximal nerve lesions are associated with greater debilitating deformity, yet this is reversed in ulnar nerve lesions as already described; this is known as the ulnar nerve paradox.

A3

a. ix – Herpes zoster. The painful vesicular lesion in a dermatomal distribution is a classical presentation of shingles. It usually affects the T3–L3 dermatomes with an erythematous maculopapular rash appearing within the first 48–72 hours that evolves into vesicular lesions. It can take up to 2–4 weeks for resolution of symptoms. The virus may affect both the motor and sensory peripheral nerves and this usually occurs 2 weeks following the dermal lesions. Nerve conduction studies typically show reduced action potential amplitude since the damage is primarily axonal.[1]

b. iv – PAN. This patient has very non-specific symptoms of generalised muscle aches and weakness. However, the skin rash described is livedo reticularis and this is a feature of PAN. It is primarily a medium vessel vasculitide and the pathophysiology is related to the production of soluble circulating immune complexes. Vascular inflammation and occlusion can lead to neuropathy in 50%–75% of people with systemic PAN.[2]

c. iii – Hypothyroidism. This lady has a classic description of CTS. Tinel's sign reproduces the pain by aggravating the median nerve. Although both hypothyroidism and diabetes are risk factors for developing CTS, this lady reports having put on weight, loss of hair and she has a bradycardia suggestive more of hypothyroidism than diabetes.

d. viii – GBS. The history suggests a distal peripheral neuropathy that ascends rapidly in keeping with GBS. GBS is an autoimmune disease caused by immune 'mimicry' where autoantibodies are produced against an antigen from a pathogen but these same autoantibodies attack the myelin on peripheral nerves. It affects motor, sensory and autonomic nerves. The paralysis ascends and can cause respiratory depression and subsequent death. Treatment is using plasma exchange or intravenous immunoglobulin, with the later usually the preferred treatment of choice. Triggers include *Campylobacter jejuni* and Epstein–Barr virus, although the flu vaccine has been linked to GBS. If progression of symptoms lasts longer than 4 weeks, the patient is then diagnosed as having chronic inflammatory demyelinating polyneuropathy.[3]

e. x – Lyme disease. The characteristic 'bullseye' rash is known as erythema migrans and usually results from a tick bite that causes an infection with *Borrelia burgdorferi*. The infection can affect the CNS and/or the peripheral nervous system usually 1–4 weeks after the tick bite. This is known as neuroborreliosis and can result in meningitis, meningoradiculitis, cranial neuritis, encephalopathy, peripheral neuropathy and encephalitis. It can even cause neuropsychiatric disorders including mania, psychosis and dementia.[4]

A4

a. x – Alcoholics are commonly deficient in vitamin B_1 (thiamine) and as a consequence are liable to develop beri beri. Dry beri beri causes peripheral nerve damage leading to the symptoms described in the vignette; wet beri beri is associated with cardiac pathology.[5]

b. i – This lady has LEMS; antibodies against voltage-gated calcium channels are highly suggestive of this diagnosis (seen in around 85% of patients). It is seen often as a paraneoplastic syndrome and presents as a more rapid MG-like syndrome accompanied with autonomic symptoms.[6]

c. vi – GBS often presents 1–3 weeks post infection as a relatively quickly ascending paralysis, unlike chronic inflammatory demyelinating polyneuropathy, which develops more slowly.[5]

d. ix – This is a case of pernicious anaemia. Prolonged vitamin B_{12} deficiency can cause subacute combined degeneration of the cord, which is a demyelinating pathology of the dorsal column and lateral corticospinal tracts.[7]

References

1. Claflin B, Thomas M, Wilson AJ. Polyradiculopathy and herpes zoster. *Proc (Bayl Univ Med Cent)*. 2009; **22**(3): 223–5.
2. Said G, Lacroix C. Primary and secondary vasculitic neuropathy. *J Neurol*. 2005; **252**(6): 633–41.
3. Hardy TA, Blum S, McCombe PA, *et al*. Guillain–Barré syndrome: modern theories of etiology. *Curr Allergy Asthma Rep*. 2011; **11**(3): 197–204.
4. Fallon BA, Levin ES, Schweitzer PJ, *et al*. Inflammation and central nervous system Lyme disease. *Neurobiol Dis*. 2010; **37**(3): 534–41.
5. Kumar P, Clark ML,editors. *Kumar & Clark's Clinical Medicine*. 7th ed. Edinburgh: Saunders Elsevier; 2009.
6. Fauci A, Braunwald E, Kasper D, *et al*., editors. *Harrison's Principles of Internal Medicine*. 17th ed. New York, NY: McGraw-Hill; 2008.
7. Goljan EF. *Rapid Review Pathology*. 3rd ed. Philadelphia, PA: Mosby/Elsevier; 2010.

16

Pathophysiology

Q1 Regarding the cells of the nervous system, which of the following statements are true and which are false?

   a. The number of neurones far exceeds the number of glial cells.

   b. Microglia are of endodermal origin.

   c. Oligodendrocytes myelinate neurones only within the CNS.

   d. One oligodendrocyte ensheaths only a single neurone thus making it vulnerable to disease.

   e. Astrocytes uptake K^+ ions from extracellular fluid following neuronal depolarisation.

Q2 Which one of the following statements concerning ependymal cells is false?

   a. Ependymal cells are simple cuboidal epithelial cells.

   b. They line the ventricles and the central canal of the spinal cord.

   c. They provide trophic support and metabolic support for progenitor cells.

   d. The choroid plexus is responsible for the re-absorption of CSF.

   e. Abnormal ependymal adhesion may lead to hydrocephalus.

Q3 An 8-year-old boy who has recently emigrated from Afghanistan visits the GP with his father. The boy presents with generalised malaise, fever and abdominal pain. He has weakness of his right leg and diminished tendon reflexes. Lumbar puncture reveals a lymphocytic infiltrate with slight elevation of protein but no changes in CSF glucose. What is the most likely microorganism that caused this boy's symptoms and findings?

a. Coronavirus

b. Coxsackievirus

c. *Campylobacter jejuni*

d. Poliovirus

e. Adenovirus

Q4 A 67-year-old woman presents to her local GP with a resting tremor, postural instability, rigidity of movement and bradykinesia. The patient is conscious and does not show any signs of decreased cognitive ability. Nervous system examination shows increased tone in the upper limbs but no sensory or proprioceptive deficits. The GP decides to start her on a drug that can also be used as an antiviral agent against influenza A. What drug has the GP most likely prescribed?

a. Bromocriptine

b. Amantadine

c. Selegiline

d. Tolcapone

e. Benztropine

Q5 A 41-year-old man with HD is prescribed haloperidol. The patient visits his GP weeks later complaining of increasing difficulty in ambulating. Vital signs include a temperature of 38.7°C, pulse rate of 124 bpm, respiratory rate of 26 breaths per minute and blood pressure of 128/82 mmHg. Laboratory test results indicate a raised serum creatine kinase. What is the most appropriate pharmacological treatment for this patient's presentation that has been caused by haloperidol?

a. Flumazenil

b. Dantrolene

c. Naloxone

d. Atropine

e. Aminocaproic acid

6 Select the microorganism that is most likely associated with each of the
following clinical scenarios.

   i. *Borrelia burgdorferi*

   ii. *Treponema pallidum*

   iii. *Mycobacterium tuberculosis*

   iv. *Mycobacterium leprae*

   v. *Bacillus anthracis*

   vi. Cytomegalovirus

   vii. Varicella zoster virus

   viii. HIV

   ix. Epstein–Barr virus

   a. A 28-year-old man presents with increased nuchal rigidity,
      disorientation and vomiting. On examination, he is positive for
      Brudzinski's and Kernig's signs. This patient is known to have
      been sexually active several years ago and had multiple partners at
      the time. Culture of his CSF reveals a heavily encapsulated yeast
      and stains positive with India ink.

   b. A person with an intact immune system contracts a disease that
      causes several skin nodules that are asymmetrically distributed
      over his body. If another person with a weak T-cell-mediated
      response contracts this same disease, the findings in this patient
      would comprise loss of eyebrows, nasal collapse and peripheral
      neuropathy. Both forms of this disease can be treated with long-
      term oral dapsone.

   c. A 41-year-old woman with HIV presents to her GP with a severe
      rash that is distributed over the T2 dermatome. After the GP
      takes a full history and examines her, he explains that these lesions
      are most likely due to a latent virus that has re-activated in her
      nerves.

   d. A 33-year-old who has been mountain climbing the previous
      weekend visits his GP because of a rash on his right leg. The rash
      resembles a 'bullseye' – it is erythematous with a central clearing.
      The GP immediately prescribes doxycycline, which effectively
      treats this patient's rash. If he were left untreated, he could
      develop a migratory polyarthritis and bilateral Bell's palsy.

e. A 46-year-old man with a known history of uncontrolled HIV presents with a painful right eye and cotton wool spots on fundoscopy. His GP explains to him that this infection exclusively occurs in immune-compromised people with a CD4 count of less than 50 per microlitre.

Q7 A 44-year-old man presents to the emergency department because he is worried about the twitching in his lips he saw while brushing his teeth – afterwards his tongue had started twitching as well. He has a 7-year history of schizophrenia. What is the usual sequence of evolution of extrapyramidal side effects from typical antipsychotics?

a. Akinesia → restlessness → tardive dyskinesia → dystonia
b. Tardive dyskinesia → restlessness → dystonia → akinesia
c. Dystonia → restlessness → akinesia → tardive dyskinesia
d. Dystonia → akinesia → restlessness → tardive dyskinesia
e. Restlessness → akinesia → tardive dyskinesia → dystonia

Q8 You are the Foundation Year 1 doctor in the A&E department. A 22-year-old man was brought in by the paramedics after he ran head first into a bus stop and fell to the ground; according to the witness he was carrying a half-empty bottle of alcohol at the time. On approaching the patient, he opens his eyes and looks at you when you ask him to, sounds like he is just stringing words together that do not make sense and withdraws from pain. You need to report your findings to your senior. What is this patient's Glasgow Coma Scale score?

a. Eye – 4, Speech – 4, Motor – 5
b. Eye – 3, Speech – 3, Motor – 4
c. Eye – 4, Speech – 3, Motor – 5
d. Eye – 4, Speech – 3, Motor – 4
e. Eye – 3, Speech – 2, Motor – 3

9 Regarding meningitis, which of the following statements are true and which are false?

   a. Meningitis usually presents with a triad of headache, neck stiffness and fever.

   b. Petechial rash is highly associated with pneumococcal infection.

   c. Brudzinski's sign is elicited by attempting passive flexion of the neck.

   d. Typical CSF changes of viral meningitis involve glucose concentrations less than half that of blood glucose.

   e. Immediate treatment for suspected meningococcal meningitis involves benzylpenicillin or, if intolerant, a tertiary cephalosporin.

10 Regarding common clinical examination signs, which of the following statements are true and which are false?

   a. Testing the bicep reflex tests the C5, C6 nerve root.

   b. The Achilles reflex tests the S4 nerve root.

   c. The Moro reflex normally disappears within the first year of life.

   d. A normal Babinski response is extensor plantar response and fanning of toes.

   e. Fasciculations are a sign of an upper motor neurone lesion.

Answers

A[1]

a. FALSE – Glial cells are 10 times more abundant than neurones. It is their ability to divide throughout life and their lack of synaptic connections that differentiate them from neurones.[1]

b. FALSE – Microglia are of mesodermal origin and responsible for the CNS immune response.[2]

   Neurones are derived from neuroectoderm.

c. TRUE – Oligodendrocytes myelinate CNS neurones and Schwann cells myelinate peripheral nervous system neurones.

d. FALSE – A single oligodendrocyte can myelinate multiple neurones and this makes it more vulnerable to disease, since the death of one oligodendrocyte will affect multiple neuronal connections. A single Schwann cell only myelinates one neurone in the peripheral nervous system.[1,3]

e. TRUE – Other functions of astrocytes include angiogenesis, structural support, neural development (through migration of neurones along radial glial cells), glycogenesis, long-term potentiation, maintenance of a blood–brain barrier, removal of neurotransmitters from synapses and the conversion of glutamate to glutamine in order for neurones to reuptake glutamine.[4,5]

A[2]

Correct answer is D – The choroid plexus is responsible for the re-absorption of CSF

During neural development, the lumen of the neural tube is lined with neural stem cells that in adults differentiate into ependymal cells lining the ventricular system. These cells are ciliated cuboidal epithelial cells, and modified ependymal cells in the lateral, third and fourth ventricles form the choroid plexus, which is responsible for the production of CSF.[6] The reabsorption of CSF is controlled by the arachnoid villi. The choroid plexus is able to modify the composition of CSF in response to events such as traumatic brain injury (e.g. releases leukocytes, growth factors and neurotrophins).[7]

A3

Correct answer is D – Poliovirus

Poliovirus, which is transmitted by the faecal-oral route, causes poliomyelitis. It is most often seen in developing countries in young unimmunised children. The virus replicates in the oropharynx and small intestine before spreading through the bloodstream to the CNS. Once in the CNS, it destroys ventral horn neurones in the spinal cord, resulting in lower motor neurone signs. A prodromal syndrome of malaise, headache, fever and abdominal pain is commonly seen. Lumbar puncture results would reveal a viral cause with no change in CSF glucose. Poliomyelitis is usually diagnosed by recovery of the virus from a stool culture.[8]

Coronavirus (answer A) causes the common cold.

Coxsackievirus (answer B) can cause aseptic meningitis, myocarditis and febrile pharyngitis. It can also cause hand, foot and mouth disease.

Campylobacter jejuni (answer C) is a major cause of bloody diarrhoea in children. Has been linked to GBS but the clinical features would be those of an ascending paralysis and not unilateral weakness.

Adenovirus (answer E) can cause febrile pharyngitis, pneumonia and conjunctivitis.

A4

Correct answer is B – Amantadine

The history and findings are typical of Parkinson's disease.[9] Amantadine is a drug that can be used in the treatment of both Parkinson's and influenza A. It blocks viral penetration as well as uncoating of the influenza virus and releases dopamine from intact nerve terminals. Since Parkinson's disease is highly associated with decreased dopamine levels, amantadine is useful in these patients. Side effects of amantadine include ataxia, dizziness and slurred speech.[10] It

should be remembered that amantadine is not a first-line drug in the tr
of Parkinson's disease.

Bromocriptine (answer A) is a dopamine receptor agonist used in th ... ...au-
ment of Parkinson's disease. It is not used as an antiviral agent.

Selegiline (answer C) selectively inhibits monoamine oxidase B therefore
increasing the availability of dopamine in Parkinson's disease. It is not used as
an antiviral agent.

Tolcapone (answer D) is a catechol-O-methyltransferase inhibitor that
prevents l-dopa degradation and therefore increases dopamine in Parkinson's
disease. It is not used as an antiviral agent.

Benztropine (answer E) is an antimuscarinic that curbs excess acetylcholine
implicated in Parkinson's disease. It is not used as an antiviral agent.

A5

Correct answer is B – Dantrolene

The fact that the man is taking haloperidol, a typical antipsychotic drug,
together with the history and findings is highly indicative of neuroleptic
malignant syndrome (NMS). NMS is a relatively rare side effect of typical antipsychotics, but it is potentially fatal. Think 'FEVER' when thinking
of patients presenting with NMS: **F**ever, **E**ncephalopathy, unstable **V**itals,
Elevated enzymes and **R**igidity of muscles. Dantrolene, which is used in the
treatment of NMS, prevents the release of Ca^{2+} from the sarcoplasmic reticu-
lum of skeletal muscle.[11]

Flumazenil (answer A) is a competitive antagonist at the GABA-A receptor.
It is used as an antidote to benzodiazepine overdose.

Naloxone (answer C) is an opioid receptor antagonist. It is used in the treatment of opioid overdose.

Atropine (answer D) is a non-selective muscarinic antagonist. It has a wide
variety of applications but not in the treatment of NMS.

Aminocaproic acid (answer E) is an inhibitor of fibrinolysis and is used to
treat toxicity caused by thrombolytics.

A6

a. viii – The initial signs and findings indicate meningitis.[12] It is also determined from the history that the man had multiple partners and had been sexually active several years ago. These risk factors are specific to sexually transmitted diseases. The additional CSF findings indicate meningitis caused by *Cryptococcus neoformans*.[13] This opportunistic fungal infection is characteristically found in patients with a low CD4 count infected with HIV.

b. iv – *Mycobacterium leprae* causes leprosy. Leprosy has two forms: tuberculoid and lepromatous. The tuberculoid form of leprosy presents with a few hypoesthetic skin nodules in patients with an intact T-cell response. However, in patients with a deficient T-cell response, lepromatous leprosy presents diffusely over the skin, infecting superficial nerves. Both types can be treated with long-term oral dapsone.[14]

c. vii – The varicella zoster virus, which causes chickenpox, most often remains dormant in the trigeminal and dorsal root ganglia long after the initial infection subsides. In the immune-compromised individual, it may reactivate in a characteristic distribution of a specific dermatome. The severe, itchy and painful rash then becomes indicative of shingles.[15]

d. i – *Borrelia burgdorferi* is a bacterium that causes Lyme disease. It is transmitted by ticks and presents with erythema chronicum migrans (expanding 'bullseye' red rash) and flu-like symptoms in its initial stages. In its later stages, patients may experience a migratory polyarthritis and bilateral Bell's palsy. Doxycycline, which is a tetracycline, is indicated for the treatment of Lyme disease.[15]

e. vi – The combination of HIV infection and cotton wool spots on fundoscopy should immediately trigger a high suspicion of retinitis caused by cytomegalovirus. This infection only occurs in severely immune-compromised people and commonly in patients with a CD4 count of less than 50 per microliter.[15]

A7

Correct answer is D – Dystonia → akinesia → restlessness → tardive dyskinesia[10]

Remember '4 DART' as a way of recalling the sequence and time delay for the usual sequence of evolution of extrapyramidal side effects from typical antipsychotics (dopamine D_2 receptor antagonists).

- **4** hours – acute **D**ystonia (muscle spasm, stiffness)
- **4** days – **A**kinesia (parkinsonian symptoms)
- **4** weeks – **R**estlessness (akathisia)
- **4** months – **T**ardive dyskinesia (oral-facial movements due to long-term use, often irreversible)

A⁸

Correct answer is B – Eye – 3, Speech – 3, Motor – 4
- Eye: 3 – opening to verbal commands
- Speech: 3 – comprehensible but consists of inappropriate words
- Motor: 4 – withdrawing from pain

The Glasgow Coma Scale gives an objective measurement of a patient's conscious level.[12]

Response	1	2	3	4	5	6
Eye	No response	To pain	To speech	Spontaneously		
Speech	No response	Incomprehensible	Inappropriate	Confused	Orientated	
Motor	No response	Extension to pain	Flexion to pain	Withdraws from pain	Localises to pain	Obeys commands

A way to remember this scale is to remember: '4-eyes', 'Jackson-5' and a '6-cylinder engine' – Eye, Speech and Motor, respectively.

A⁹

a. TRUE – This triad is highly suggestive of a meningitic syndrome; photophobia and vomiting are also often present.
b. FALSE – A petechial rash is highly associated with a meningococcal infection.
c. TRUE – Kernig's and Brudzinski's signs usually appear within hours:
   - **K**ernig's – pain elicited on leg extension at the **K**nee when the hip is flexed
   - Brudzinski's – pain elicited on passive neck flexion.

d. FALSE – In viral meningitis, the CSF to serum glucose ratio is usually normal but can be elevated, not decreased. Protein count can be increased and the white blood cell (WBC) count low. High protein levels in the CSF combined with a decreased CSF to serum glucose ratio and raised opening pressures would be highly suggestive of a bacterial meningitis. *See* the table provided following outlining the characteristic CSF changes in meningitis of different aetiologies.[12]

Aetiology	Protein	Glucose content	Appearance	Other
Normal	–	60% of serum glucose	Clear	–
Bacterial	Mild to moderate elevation	Usually decreased	Turbid/Purulent	Raised WBC count Opening pressure raised Increased polymorphonucleocytes
Viral	Normal to elevated	Usually normal	Clear/Turbid	WBC count usually low Early phase – mostly neutrophils Late phase – mostly lymphocytes
Tuberculosis	Elevated	Decreased	Turbid/Viscous	Increased lymphocytes
Fungal	Elevated	Decreased	Turbid/Viscous	Increased lymphocytes

e. TRUE – Antibiotics may be given empirically and up to 2 hours before a lumbar puncture is performed.

A 10

a. TRUE – Testing the bicep reflex does test the C5, C6 nerve root.
b. FALSE – S1, S2 are tested in the Achilles reflex. Major reflexes 'count up' as they 'go up' the body:
   - S1, S2 – Achilles
   - L3, L4 – patellar
   - C5, C6 – biceps
   - C7, C8 – triceps.
c. TRUE – The Moro reflex is the rapid abduction followed by adduction of limbs when startled. It normally disappears within the first year of

life and may re-emerge following frontal lobe lesions, along with other primitive reflexes.[12] The primitive reflexes can be remembered using 'MRS BP':

- **M**oro
- **R**ooting (movement of head towards side of cheek/mouth that is stroked)
- **S**ucking (sucking response when the roof of the mouth is touched)
- **B**abinski's sign
- **P**almar and **P**lantar (curling of digits when the palmar surfaces of hands or feet are stroked).

d. FALSE – This is an *abnormal* Babinski response, the normal response is for flexion of toes.[12]

e. FALSE – Fasciculations are a sign of lower motor neurone lesions.

Sign	Upper motor neurone lesion	Lower motor neurone lesion
Weakness	+	+
Atrophy	−	+
Fasciculations	−	+
Reflexes	↑	↓
Tone	↑	↓

References

1. Siegel GJ, Agranoff BW, Albers RW, *et al. Basic Neurochemistry: molecular, cellular, and medical aspects*. Philadelphia, PA: Lippincott Williams & Wilkins; 1999.
2. Long-Smith CM, Sullivan AM, Nolan YM. The influence of microglia on the pathogenesis of Parkinson's disease. *Prog Neurobiol*. 2009; **89**(3): 277–87.
3. Shephard GM. *Neurobiology*. New York, NY: Oxford University Press; 1994.
4. Slezak M, Pfrieger FW, Soltys Z. Synaptic plasticity, astrocytes and morphological homeostasis. *J Physiol Paris*. 2006; **99**(2–3): 84–91.
5. Freeman MR. Sculpting the nervous system: glial control of neuronal development. *Curr Opin Neurobiol*. 2006; **16**(1): 119–25.
6. Carlén M, Meletis K, Göritz C, *et al.* Forebrain ependymal cells are Notch-dependent and generate neuroblasts and astrocytes after stroke. *Nat Neurosci*. 2009; **12**(3): 259–67.
7. Johanson C, Stopa E, Baird A, *et al.* Traumatic brain injury and recovery mechanisms: peptide modulation of periventricular neurogenic regions by the choroid plexus-CSF nexus. *J Neural Transm*. 2011; **118**(1): 115–33.

8. Frosch MP, Anthony DC, De Girolami U. The central nervous system. In: Kumar V, Abbas AK, Fausto N, *et al. Robbins and Cotran Pathologic Basis of Disease, Professional Edition*. 8th ed. Philadelphia, PA: Saunders Elsevier; 2010.
9. Bowker LK, Price JD, Smith SC. Neurology. *Oxford Handbook of Geriatric Medicine*. Oxford: Oxford University Press; 2006. pp. 163–90.
10. Rang HP, Dale MM, Ritter JM, *et al*. Neurodegenerative diseases. *Rang and Dale's Pharmacology*. 6th ed. New York, NY: Churchill Livingstone; 2007. p. 512.
11. Burke C, Fulda GJ, Castellano J. Neuroleptic malignant syndrome in a trauma patient. *J Trauma*. 1995; **39**(4): 796–8.
12. Kumar PJ, Clark ML, editors. *Kumar & Clark's Clinical Medicine*. 7th ed. Edinburgh: Saunders Elsevier; 2009.
13. Schneider AS, Szanto PA. Respiratory system. *Pathology*. Philadelphia, PA: Wolters Kluwer Health/Lippincott Williams & Wilkins; 2009. p. 207.
14. Mahan S. Mycobacterium. In: Gladwin M, Trattler B. *Clinical Microbiology Made Ridiculously Simple*. 5th ed. Miami, FL: MedMaster; 2011. pp. 147–53.
15. McAdam AJ, Sharpe AH. Infectious diseases. In: Kumar V, Abbas AK, Fausto N, *et al. Robbins and Cotran Pathologic Basis of Disease, Professional Edition*. 8th ed. Philadelphia, PA: Elsevier; 2010. pp. 353–5, 377–8.

17

Radiculopathies

Q1 Jonathan presents to his GP as he has been experiencing some odd symptoms. He finds it very difficult to flex the fingers of his right hand. On neurological examination, he can shrug his shoulders, has normal elbow flexion and extension and normal wrist power. However, his grip strength on the right is noticeably reduced. The GP suspects Jonathan is suffering from a pinched nerve. Which nerve root is most likely to be affected?

a. C5

b. C6

c. C7

d. C8

e. T1

Q2 A 32-year-old tennis player presents to his GP with a 4-week history of progressive neck and right arm discomfort accompanied by numbness on the lateral aspect of the right forearm and thumb, with weakness of elbow flexion. Shoulder abduction is normal. There are no symptoms in the lower limbs, and no bladder or bowel disturbance. He has no significant medical history and is otherwise well. There is no history of significant trauma.

Select the most likely cause for his symptoms from the following.
a. Radial nerve injury
b. C6 nerve root compression
c. CTS
d. Diabetic peripheral neuropathy

Q3 A 55-year-old woman presents to her GP with low back pain for the past 4 weeks accompanied by shooting pains down the lateral aspect of her left thigh and into the dorsal aspect of her left foot. The pain does not keep her up at night, is located in the lumbar region and there are no bladder or bowel symptoms. She feels otherwise well and has not lost weight.

Select the most likely cause of her symptoms from the following.
a. Spondyloarthropathy
b. Spinal tumour
c. Diabetic neuropathy
d. Muscular spasm

Q^4

PART A

Label the parts of the lumbar vertebra shown below, a–f

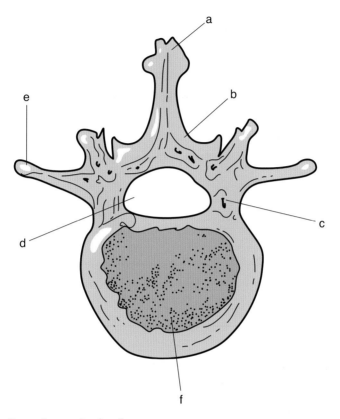

 i. Superior articular facet
 ii. Inferior articular facet
 iii. Transverse process
 iv. Spinous process
 v. Pedicle
 vi. Vertebral body
 vii. Mammillary process
 viii. Lamina
 ix. Spinal canal

PART B

A 25-year-old man complains of ongoing back pain for the past month. He is a gymnast who trains at least three times a week. The pain is located in the lumbosacral area and is much worse after activity. On examination, he is unable to straight leg raise his right leg more than 40 degrees because of pain in the posterior compartment of his thigh. Lasegue's and Bragard's tests are positive. The patient also has reduced sensation in the posterior-lateral aspect of his leg with weakness in ankle plantarflexion. What is the level of his radiculopathy?

a. L3

b. L4

c. L5

d. S1

e. S2

Answers

A[1]

Correct answer is D – C8

The myotome for finger flexion is C8. The upper limb myotomes are as follows.[1]
- Shoulder abduction – C5
- Shoulder adduction – C6, C7, C8
- Elbow flexion – C5, C6 (biceps)
- Elbow extension – C6, C7 (triceps)
- Wrist extension – C6
- Wrist flexion – C7
- Finger extension – C7
- Finger flexion – C8
- Finger abduction/adduction – T1

A[2]

Correct answer is B – C6 nerve root compression

In this case, the symptoms fit best with a C6 nerve root compression. Radial nerve injury would commonly consist of wrist drop and numbness of the dorsal surface of the hand, mainly of the anatomical snuffbox. The C6 nerve innervates the lateral aspect of the arm and thumb and is responsible for elbow flexion and forearm pronation and supination. CTS affects the median nerve as it passes through the carpal tunnel, thus usually only affecting sensation in the thumb and first two fingers of the hand and affecting motor function in most notably the abductor pollicis brevis.[1] Diabetic peripheral neuropathy is more common in older patients and is unlikely in a young patient with no history of diabetes.[2]

A³

Correct answer is A – Spondyloarthropathy

This woman has an L5 radiculopathy, evidenced by the L5 dermatomal pattern of the pain. Other signs associated with this are weakness of toe extension and ankle inversion or eversion may be affected.[1] Spondyloarthropathy is the most common cause of lumbosacral radiculopathy, along with disc disease.[3] Other causes include multiple myeloma, metastatic spinal tumours, spinal infections such as vertebral osteomyelitis and spinal cord tumours such as spinal cord meningiomas, although all of these are rare.[4]

A⁴

PART A

a. iv – Spinous process
b. viii – Lamina
c. v – Pedicle
d. ix – Spinal canal
e. iii – Transverse process
f. vi – Vertebral body

PART B

Correct answer is D – S1

The man is suffering from compression of the S1 nerve root and this is characterised by the distribution of his reduced sensation and weakness in ankle plantarflexion. The straight leg raise test reproduces his pain by stretching the sciatic nerve, which has roots from L4 to S3.

Take a look at the Apparelyzed website (www.apparelyzed.com/dermatome.html), an online spinal cord injury peer support forum. It has several diagrams of dermatomes and it also has an excellent reference list of how to test each dermatome clinically (e.g. testing sensation over the lateral ante-cubital fossa tests the C5 dermatome).

References

1. Crossman AR, Neary D. *Neuroanatomy: an illustrated colour text*. 3rd ed. Ediburgh: Elsevier; 2005.
2. Young MJ, Boulton AJ, MacLeod AF, *et al*. A multicentre study of the prevalence of diabetic peripheral neuropathy in the United Kingdom hospital clinic population. *Diabetologia*. 1993; **36**(2): 150–4.
3. Tarulli AW, Raynor EM. Lumbosacral radiculopathy. *Neurol Clin*. 2007; **25**(2): 387–405.
4. Shelerud RA, Paynter KS. Rarer causes of radiculopathy: spinal tumours, infections, and other unusual causes. *Phys Med Rehabil Clin N Am*. 2002; **13**(3): 645–96.

18
Spinal cord lesions

Q1   A 60-year-old man presents to his GP with 2 months of progressive back pain, located in the lower thoracic spine, which despite ibuprofen and paracetamol, prevents him from sleeping at night when the pain is worst. He worked until recently as a builder. He has noticed that he has lost weight over the past few months despite an increasingly sedentary lifestyle. He gave up smoking 2 years ago but has a 30 pack year history and has had a non-productive cough for the last year. Which of the following is the most appropriate management?

    a.   Referral for physiotherapy

    b.   Routine referral to spinal surgeon

    c.   Urgent referral for spinal and chest imaging

    d.   Increase pain relief, review in 1 month

Q2   Regarding lesions of the spinal cord, which of the following statements are true and which are false?

    a.   Autonomic function is always preserved.

    b.   In acute compression there will be spasticity in muscles below the level of the lesion.

    c.   The commonest cause of cord compression is intervertebral disc prolapse.

    d.   A spinal MRI scan is essential

    e.   In Brown-Séquard's syndrome, there is ipsilateral loss of proprioception and vibration, and contralateral loss of pain and temperature.

Q3 Select the correct cause or diagnosis associated with the types of spinal cord lesions highlighted in the cross-section diagram shown below. Each answer may be selected more than once.

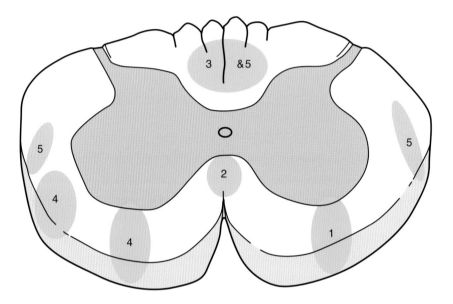

  i. Werdnig–Hoffmann disease
 ii. MS
iii. ALS
 iv. Occlusion of the anterior spinal artery
  v. Tabes dorsalis
 vi. Syringomyelia
vii. Vitamin B_{12} neuropathy
viii. Brown-Séquard's syndrome
 ix. Sturge–Weber syndrome

a. 1
b. 2
c. 3
d. 4
e. 5

Answers

A[1]

Correct answer is C – Urgent referral for spinal and chest imaging

This man has presented with a number of 'red flag' symptoms of back pain. The red flag symptoms in this case are thoracic back pain, age over 55, nocturnal pain and unintentional weight loss.[1] Because of his extensive smoking history and worrying-sounding cough, an urgent referral is appropriate to investigate potential spinal metastases, as well as to look for a possible lung primary. Prostate, breast, lung, kidney, thyroid tumours and melanomas most commonly metastasize to bone.

A[2]

a. FALSE – It is vital to ask about autonomic dysfunction in patients with back pain or back injury. In cauda equina (which is a medical emergency) where there is compression of a number of spinal nerves, there may be urinary/bowel incontinence or painless retention or erectile dysfunction. In those with high spinal cord injuries, for example, patients may have difficulty regulating blood pressure, heart rate and sweating. Hence, a tetraplegic patient after a cervical cord injury may suffer with brady-arrhythmias and erratic blood pressures.

b. FALSE – Patients presenting with acute cord compression will not immediately show upper motor neurone signs below the level of the spinal cord lesion. Thus, initially there will be reduced tone and diminished reflexes (spinal shock). This will later progress to spasticity and hyperreflexia as the interneurones in the CNS begin to increase synaptic connections. At the level of the cord compression, there will be lower motor neurones signs, and above the lesion the patient should be asymptomatic.

c. FALSE – The commonest cause is secondary metastases from the lung, breast and prostate. Other, rarer, causes include epidural abscess, haematomas (in particular, in patients receiving warfarin) and spinal cord tumours.

d. TRUE – Plain X-rays have a limited use in these patients but MRI is the gold standard. All of the causes listed in the previous paragraph can be detected using MRI. If a mass is detected then further surgical management may be required.

e. TRUE
   - Below the level of the Brown-Séquard lesion:
     ‣ corticospinal tract damage causes ipsilateral weakness, spasticity, hyperreflexia and positive Babinski sign
     ‣ dorsal column damage causes ipsilateral loss of proprioception, vibration and discriminative touch
     ‣ spinothalamic tract damage causes contralateral loss of light touch, pressure, pain and temperature.
   - At the level of the Brown-Séquard lesion:
     ‣ damage to the ventral horns causes ipsilateral muscle weakness with flaccid paralysis and hyporeflexia.

Upper motor neurone lesions	Lower motor neurone lesions
Weakness in extensor muscles of the arm and flexor muscles of the leg	Muscles supplied by the affected peripheral nerve will be weakened
Spasticity (increased muscle tone) in flexor muscles of the arm and extensor muscles of the leg	Hypotonia (decreased muscle tone) in affected muscles
Very little muscle wasting	Muscles may show wasting
Hyperreflexia	Reflexes are reduced
Babinski sign positive (up-going plantars)	Babinski sign is negative
Presence of clonus	There may be fasciculation

A3

a. i – The location indicated here shows a lesion in the ventral horn region of the spinal cord which contains bodies of lower motor neurones. Of all the answers given, Werdnig–Hoffmann disease is the only answer on the list that is characterised as involving lesions in the lower motor neurones of the spinal cord and degeneration of ventral horns. This disease presents at birth as a 'floppy baby' and displays an autosomal recessive pattern of inheritance.[2]

b. vi – Syringomyelia (collection of CSF in the central canal) can lead to damage of the anterior white commissure of the spinothalamic tract (located close to the central canal), which results in bilateral loss of pain and temperature sensation. Proprioception and vibration senses carried by dorsal column tracts are unaffected. Syringomyelia most commonly occurs at the vertebral level C8–T1 and is seen with Arnold–Chiari types 1 and 2.

c. v – Tabes dorsalis occurs because of the degeneration of dorsal columns and is seen in tertiary syphilis. As a result, impaired proprioception and locomotor ataxia are evident in these patients. Other symptoms and findings associated with tabes dorsalis include Argyll Robertson pupils (reactive to accommodation but not to light), a positive Romberg's sign and sensory ataxia at night.

d. iii – ALS affects the lateral corticospinal tract and ventral horn. Characteristic findings include upper and lower motor neurone signs but with the absence of sensory or cognitive deficits.

e. vii – Vitamin B_{12} neuropathy (subacute combined degeneration of the cord) is a relatively common condition among older people. Demyelination of dorsal columns, lateral corticospinal tracts and spinocerebellar tracts occur. Findings include an ataxic gait, dementia, loss of discriminative touch and pressure, and impaired position and vibration sense. Non-neurological findings include a megaloblastic anaemia (B_{12} deficiency is associated with pernicious anaemia where there is a loss of gastric parietal cells) and glossitis.[3]

References

1. Speed C. Low back pain. *BMJ*. 2004; **328**(7448): 1119–21.
2. Anthony DC, Frosch MP, De Girolami U. Peripheral nerve and skeletal muscle. In: Kumar V, Abbas AK, Fausto N, *et al. Robbins and Cotran Pathologic Basis of Disease, Professional Edition*. 8th ed. Philadelphia, PA: Saunders Elsevier; 2010. pp. 1267–8.
3. Frosch MP, Anthony DC, De Girolami U. The central nervous system. In: Kumar V, Abbas AK, Fausto N, *et al. Robbins and Cotran Pathologic Basis of Disease, Professional Edition*. 8th ed. Philadelphia, PA: Saunders Elsevier; 2010.

19

Stroke

Q1 A 62-year-old man was brought in by his wife to the A&E department an hour after suddenly collapsing on his way home from town. He recalls having experienced right-sided arm and leg weakness and slurred speech before collapsing and there was no loss of consciousness. The gentleman is a known diabetic. Following a plain brain CT scan, the man was given thrombolysis. He went on to develop expressive dysphasia. Select from the following list what he was diagnosed with.

a. Posterior circulation stroke
b. Severe migraine
c. Partial anterior circulation infarct
d. Partial anterior circulation haemorrhage
e. Lacunar infarct

Q2 Regarding cerebral strokes, which of the following statements are true and which are false?

a. Posterior cerebral artery occlusion causes contralateral homonymous hemianopia.
b. Unilateral vasospasm of the anterior cerebral artery will primarily cause weakness of the ipsilateral leg.
c. Haemorrhagic stroke is far more prevalent than ischaemic stroke.
d. Atrial fibrillation is the most significant risk factor for the development of ischaemic stroke.
e. Pure motor hemiparesis can result from infarction of the lenticulo-striatal arteries.

Q3 A 75-year-old woman was found by her daughter collapsed on the floor and unable to move her left arm and leg. She had been lying there for several hours. Upon hospital admission and on examination, she was hypothermic with a blood pressure of 180/110 mmHg, a pulse of 95 bpm and oxygen saturation of 93% on air. The left arm and leg are flaccid and her mouth is drooping on the left side. Following her admission, which of the following investigations must be carried out immediately?

a. Blood glucose level

b. Echocardiogram

c. CT scan

d. MRI

e. Carotid Doppler scan

Q4 Concerning strokes and transient ischaemic attacks, which of the following statements are true and which are false?

a. The salvageable area surrounding an infarction is known as the penumbra.

b. Amaurosis fugax is sudden-onset transient monocular blindness due to retinal artery occlusion.

c. The lenticulostriate arteries arise from the anterior cerebral artery.

d. A stroke involving the middle cerebral artery is likely to produce aphasia.

e. During the acute management of a stroke, achieving a normal blood pressure is of importance.

Q5   With regard to strokes, match each of the clinical signs to the most likely lesion. Answers may be used more than once.

    i.   Anterior cerebral artery

    ii.   Posterior inferior cerebellar artery

    iii.   Anterior choroidal artery

    iv.   Posterior communicating artery

    v.   Basilar artery

    vi.   Posterior cerebral artery

    vii.   Anterior inferior cerebellar artery

    viii.   Middle cerebral artery

    ix.   Superior cerebellar artery

    x.   Anterior inferior cerebellar artery

    a.   Wernicke's aphasia

    b.   'Locked-in' syndrome

    c.   Unilateral lower limb paresis

    d.   Cortical blindness

    e.   Lateral medullary syndrome

Q6   After an ischaemic stroke, a 71-year-old patient is found to have a complete change in personality. He is constantly putting things in his mouth even though he is not hungry. The nurses also note that he gets sudden sexual urges, which they deem as highly inappropriate. His behaviour appears to be completely uninhibited. A diagnosis of Klüver–Bucy syndrome is made. Where is the lesion most likely located?

    a.   PPRF

    b.   Bilateral mammillary bodies

    c.   Right parietal lobe

    d.   Bilateral amygdala

    e.   Basal ganglia

Q7

i. Hypoglossal dysarthria

ii. Dysnomia

iii. Hoarseness

iv. Speech dyspraxia

v. Broca's dysphasia

vi. Wernicke's dysphasia

vii. Conduction aphasia

viii. Global aphasia

ix. Facial dysarthria

The following patients present with problems with their speech and language. They are right-handed. Please select the most accurate option(s) from the list to answer each of the following questions. Each option may be used once or more than once.

a. A 58-year-old man suffers a stroke. Although he can *understand* speech well, his replies do not make sense. He also has weakness in his right arm and face.

b. A 60-year-old woman is walking in the park when her husband notices her speech has suddenly become confusing. She's brought to the A&E department where you see her. She can't seem to follow your commands and, on top of the collateral history, you notice her speech is fluent but makes no sense.

c. A 55-year-old smoker comes to you explaining his recent voice change. He says he has been losing weight for the past few months. He also says he can't walk as far as he used to and needs to stop to catch his breath.

d. A man suffers a head injury for which he is treated and looked after in the A&E department. Following the trauma he is fit and his speech is understandable but he seems to have trouble with 'la' sounds.

e. You need to see a 51-year-old woman to test for a suspected speech complication due to a trauma to the head. You examine her and assess that she can follow three-stage commands but cannot seem to name common objects such as a pen; she communicates what the name of the object is by grabbing the pen off you and writing it down.

Q^8

   i. Total anterior circulation infarction

   ii. Partial anterior circulation infarction

  iii. Lacunar infarction

  iv. Posterior circulation infarction

   v. Syncope

  vi. Infective endocarditis

 vii. Ruptured berry aneurysm

viii. Mural thrombus

  ix. Vertigo

   x. Paradoxical emboli

For the following questions, please choose from the answers listed. The answers may be used once or more than once. The patients are all right-hand dominant. What is the most accurate diagnosis in each case?

a. A 57-year-old teacher with a medical history of hypertension presents after waking up and falling a few feet away from his bed because the 'room was spinning around him'. He remembers it clearly as this is the first time it has happened. He complains of seeing double, and on finger-to-nose testing, you notice a tremor when he extends his hand and he finds it difficult to touch your finger.

b. A 39-year-old man is brought to the A&E department by his friends from the bar, where he thought someone hit him over the head with a bottle. His feet hang off the end of the bed and you notice his long fingers and slender physique. He has a Glasgow Coma Scale score of 13 with a severe headache and no signs of trauma.

c. You see a 72-year-old lady on the ward, several days after her initial collapse. When asking for consent to perform a peripheral neurological exam, she does not respond and you notice her hearing aids. You think the batteries are dead so you step over to her left-hand side and ask again. She is still having a hard time hearing you, she articulates with difficulty and in the end she nods. On examination, you assess that she has weakness in her right arm and leg alongside some sensory loss.

d. A 22-year-old man with a history of anaemia presented with a fever yesterday. You are the Foundation Year 1 doctor and find him with his arm hanging off the bed and that he has developed a new-onset left-sided weakness in his face and arms. You remember that when you examined him, you noticed a new murmur over his mitral valve, his yellow teeth, halitosis and peculiar small, painful raised lesions on his palms.

e. You meet a 61-year-old manager who comes into the A&E department with facial weakness and problems with his speech. He has a Glasgow Coma Scale score of 12 and you can hear bi-basal crackles in his lungs. He had a heart attack recently, and in the notes, his previous electrocardiogram tracing showed an anterior wall myocardial infarction.

Q9 A 66-year-old man with hypertension has been vomiting but is not sure whether it is due to the headache he is having on the back of his head or his sudden dizziness. Examination reveals a nystagmus to the left, and hypotonia and hyporeflexia of his left-sided limbs. His heart rate is regular at 78 bpm with a blood pressure of 210/105 mmHg. The results of a CT scan of his head show changes in his left cerebellar peduncle.

a. Cerebellar infarction

b. Alcohol excess

c. Hypothyroidism

d. Vertigo

e. Cerebellopontine angle tumour

Q10 A 58-year-old man with a 10-year history of hypertension and diabetes suffers a collapse in the morning. His blood glucose levels are 7 mmol, HbA$_{1C}$ is 5.5% and he has a blood pressure of 129/76 mmHg. In the evening he seems well, but on peripheral neurological examination you notice decreased power in his right arm and leg; however, he can still sense pinpricks and cotton wool over these areas. He also seems to be using his left hand to wipe the drool off the right side of his mouth. What is the most likely diagnosis?

a. Infarct of the right internal capsule

b. Infarct of the left internal capsule

c. Infarct of the right thalamus

d. Infarct of the left thalamus

e. Trauma from a hypoglycaemic fall

Answers

A¹

Correct answer is C – Partial anterior circulation infarct

This man's old age, diabetic medical history and focal neurological signs favour the diagnosis of acute stroke in this case, as opposed to severe migraine. The fact that the man was thrombolysed following a plain CT brain scan means that the stroke was ischaemic rather than haemorrhagic.[1] In this case, it is a partial anterior circulation infarct since he has dysphasia (higher dysfunction) as well as arm and leg weakness. If he had a homonymous hemianopia also, the diagnosis would favour a total anterior circulation infarct. It is important to keep in mind that hemiplegic migraine can present like a stroke and must also not be confused with a transient ischaemic attack (TIA).

A posterior circulation stroke can be ruled out, as this would present with a variety of unique symptoms such as cerebellar dysfunction and nystagmus.[2] A lacunar infarct would not cause expressive dysphasia, which would require damage to the dominant left temporal lobe.[3]

A²

a. TRUE – The posterior cerebral artery is formed from the bifurcation of the basilar artery and supplies the midbrain, thalamus, occipital lobes, inferior aspects of the temporal lobes and inferior aspects of the parietal lobes. Patients usually develop a contralateral homonymous hemianopia (frequently with macular sparing).[4]

b. FALSE – It will cause weakness predominantly in the contralateral leg and may affect the contralateral arm (more mildly). The anterior cerebral artery supplies the frontal and medial aspects of the cerebral hemispheres (refer to the motor homunculus if unfamiliar). If both arteries are infarcted, an akinetic mutism may result where the patient is unable to speak or move as a result of severe frontal lobe damage.[5]

c. FALSE – Ischaemic stroke accounts for approximately 84% of all strokes, of which the majority are thrombotic rather than embolic events.

d. FALSE – Atrial fibrillation *is* a major risk factor; however, the most significant modifiable risk factor is hypertension. This is thought to be a result of the vascular remodelling which occurs with hypertension and the subsequent development of atherosclerosis and lipohyalinosis. Other modifiable risk factors for stroke include diabetes, congestive heart failure, smoking and hypercholesterolaemia.[6] Age is the single most important non-modifiable risk factor for stroke.

e. TRUE – The lenticulostriatal arteries arise from the middle cerebral artery and supply the internal capsule and caudate nucleus. Infarction of these small arteries causes what is known as a lacunar infarct. This can result in five common syndromes: pure motor hemiparesis, pure sensory stroke, mixed sensorimotor, ataxic hemiparesis and clumsy hand dysarthria syndrome.

A3

a. TRUE – If this patient's blood glucose were low, this could result in a seizure causing unilateral weakness (Todd's paralysis). A resolution of function may be achieved by correcting the hypoglycaemia.

b. FALSE – An echocardiogram would not be a first-line investigation in a stroke patient. It would not change the acute management; if there was no haemorrhage on the CT scan, and the patient presented within 3 hours, then they would still be a candidate for thrombolysis regardless of the echocardiogram. The echocardiogram may be useful at a later date, once the patient is stable from a neurological point of view, to assess left ventricular function/assess any new murmurs.

c. TRUE – A CT scan within the first 48 hours provides very good resolution for blood and this can help to differentiate between an ischaemic and a haemorrhagic stroke. After 48 hours, the sensitivity for haemorrhagic and ischaemic strokes begins to decrease, and this is when an MRI scan could be considered. For this reason, a CT scan should be performed as soon as possible if a patient is suspected of having had a stroke. A CT scan is *urgently* needed if a patient presents within 3 hours and may be suitable for thrombolysis.

d. FALSE – MRI scans are expensive and time consuming. The gold standard is a CT head in the first 3 hours to rule out a haemorrhagic stroke. MRI scans are more useful for delayed presentations of stroke usually after 48 hours.

e. FALSE – A carotid Doppler scan would be performed if stenosis of the carotid arteries were suspected. However, in the patient's current condition, even if a stenosis were found, a carotid endarterectomy would not be possible. Once the patient is stable and an ischaemic stroke is confirmed then a carotid Doppler may be requested.

A4

a. TRUE – The penumbra is the ischaemic zone around an area of infarction that has not yet undergone irreversible cellular changes.[7]

b. TRUE – Amaurosis fugax is associated with transient ischaemic attacks and is often described as a 'curtain' or 'veil'-like loss of vision.[1]

c. FALSE – The lenticulostriate arteries branch from the middle cerebral artery.[7]

d. TRUE – Aphasias are often seen with middle cerebral artery strokes.[7]

e. FALSE – Preserving cerebral perfusion is critical; lowering blood pressure to a normotensive range in the acute setting is likely to impede this.[8] Further care must be taken in hypertensive patients on medications for their blood pressure because if they usually have a higher blood pressure reading then even a systolic pressure which would be normal for a non-hypertensive patient may be very hypotensive for the hypertensive patient on treatment.

A5

a. viii – The middle cerebral artery supplies Wernicke's area via the angular artery and posterior parietal artery.[9]

b. v – A basilar artery lesion that prevents blood flow to the pons may result in 'locked-in' syndrome: almost complete paralysis sparing only ocular muscles supplied by cranial nerve III. The cortex is preserved and therefore no cognitive impairment is seen.[1]

c. i – The anterior cerebral artery supplies the medial aspect of the motor cortex, thereby supplying the area of the motor cortex that controls movement of the lower limb.[7]

d. vi – The posterior cerebral artery gives off the calcarine arteries, which supply most of the visual cortex. Occlusion of the distal posterior cerebral artery produces cortical blindness (blindness with pupillary reflex preservation).[11]

e. ii – Lateral medullary syndrome (vertigo, cerebellar and sensory signs, Horner's syndrome and dysphagia) arises as a result of occlusion of the posterior inferior cerebellar artery (or vertebral occlusion).[1]

A6

Correct answer is D – Bilateral amygdala

Klüver–Bucy syndrome presents with the clinical triad of hyperorality, hypersexuality and disinhibited behaviour. An ischaemic stroke, encephalitis and Alzheimer's disease can cause it. The location of the lesion responsible for this presentation is the amygdala (bilateral lesion), which is involved in memory, emotion and sexuality. Although a relatively uncommon condition, it is important to distinguish it from other lesions that may present similarly.[10]

The PPRF (answer A) is involved in the sleep–wake cycle. A lesion here would present with the patient looking away from the side of the lesion (contralateral gaze deviation). A bilateral PPRF lesion would cause a horizontal gaze palsy.

A lesion in the bilateral mammillary bodies (answer B) would result in Wernicke–Korsakoff syndrome as a result of thiamine deficiency.

A lesion in the right parietal lobe (answer C) would result in spatial neglect syndrome.

A lesion in the basal ganglia (answer E) may result in tremor at rest, chorea or athetosis.

A7

a. v – This man has had a stroke in the posterior inferior frontal lobe. This has led to non-fluent, agrammatic speech (expressive dysphasia). Due to the proximity of the primary motor cortex to the Broca's area, there is associated weakness in the face and arm.[1,9]

Remember: '**B**roken **B**roca's'

b. vi – This woman has had a stroke in the posterior superior temporal lobe. The combination of nonsensical speech and lack of comprehension is typical of a Wernicke's dysphasia or 'sensory or receptive' dysphasia.[1,9]

Remember: '**W**ordy **W**ernicke's'

c. iii – He is explaining his symptoms to you, meaning that his higher speech functions are normal and the change in the patient's voice is hoarseness. This is could be due to a cancer in his lung affecting the recurrent laryngeal nerve acting on his vocal cords.[1]

d. i – This man has cranial nerve XII (hypoglossal) weakness leading to dysarthria due to an inability to make 'la' sounds. Other sounds to note are 'kuh' for palate elevation in testing the vagus, and 'mi' in testing the lips and facial nerve. This is a more accurate diagnosis than facial dysarthria.

Remember: '**Kuh**La**M**ity' (calamity)[1]

e. ii – This woman has dysnomia: an inability to name objects such as the pen despite all other functioning being normal. This is a tricky language disorder to determine because patients may hide their inability; therefore, a Mini-Mental State Examination is a useful tool in assessing this function.

A[8]

a. iv – The patient has cerebellar signs of ataxia and an intention tremor. Other cerebellar findings could include nystagmus and dysarthria. He also has vertigo, which can be associated with posterior circulation stroke. Other features of posterior circulation stroke may include a homonymous hemianopia, contralateral sensory deficit and/or contralateral motor deficit (*see* Table 1).[1,11]

b. vii – His physical features are suggestive of a person with Marfan's syndrome, which has a predisposition to causing berry aneurysms. Aneurysms are also associated with adult polycystic kidney disease and Ehlers–Danlos syndrome. His symptoms of a severe headache and no signs of trauma are highly indicative of a SAH caused by a ruptured aneurysm.[12]

c. i – The lady in this case has been deaf for a while, given the presence of hearing aids; the fact that she responds after you move to a different side (alongside her other symptoms of presentation) should alert you to the possibility of a homonymous hemianopia. She is having trouble with her speech alongside reduced movement and sensation in her right-side limbs. The triad of defects are the result of a 'total' anterior circulation stroke; if she only had two of the three symptoms, she would have had a partial anterior circulation stroke (*see* Table 1).[1,11]

d. vi – Infective endocarditis can cause septic emboli to dislodge, most commonly from the mitral valve (highest pressure), resulting in stroke. Poor teeth hygiene is associated with a risk of developing infective endocarditis. Infective endocarditis is usually caused by *Streptococcus viridans* (having a more insidious onset) and *Staphylococcus aureus* (most common in intravenous drug users). Fever, anaemia, new murmur (valvular damage) and Osler's nodes on the palms are highly suggestive of the diagnosis.[1]

> Remember: 'FROM JANE'
> - **F**ever
> - **R**oth's spots (**R**etina)
> - **O**sler's nodes (**O**uch – are painful)
> - **M**urmur (**M**itral)
> - **J**aneway lesion (**J**arred loose – septic emboli)
> - **A**naemia
> - **N**ail-bed haemorrhages
> - **E**mboli

e. viii – The anterior wall myocardial infarction most likely led to a left ventricular aneurysm and possible intraventricular thrombus in the heart wall. The differential of an arrhythmia as the aetiology is still possible; however, the risk is highest within 2–4 days, as opposed to ventricular aneurysm and subsequent mural thrombus, which is the most likely complication at any point >7 weeks post-myocardial infarction. Paradoxical emboli would originate in the right side of the heart. Paradoxical emboli are usually from a lower limb venous thrombus that passes through a septal defect into the left side of the heart and into the systemic circulation.[1]

TABLE 1 Oxford (Bamford) classification of stroke

Type of stroke and affected territory	Symptoms and signs
Total anterior circulation infarction (TACI): usually at the level of the middle cerebral artery or internal carotid artery	All **three 'H's**: • **h**igher cerebral dysfunction (e.g. dysphasia, dyscalculia) • **h**omonymous hemianopia • **h**emiparesis/hemisensory loss affecting at least two body areas
Partial anterior circulation infarction (PACI): more restricted cortical infarcts in the distribution of the middle and anterior cerebral arteries	• Only **two of three 'H'** components of the total anterior circulation stroke or • Motor/Sensory deficit restricted to face or arm or leg
Posterior circulation infarction (POCI): compromised blood flow in the posterior cerebral arteries or vertebrobasilar system affecting the brainstem, cerebellum and occipital lobes	• Ipsilateral cranial nerve palsy with contralateral motor and/or sensory deficit • Bilateral motor and/or sensory deficit • Disorder of conjugate eye movement • Cerebellar dysfunction without ipsilateral hemiparesis • Isolated homonymous hemianopia
Lacunar infarction: small infarcts in the basal ganglia or internal capsule	• Pure motor, pure sensory or mixed sensory-motor deficit • Ataxic hemiparesis

A[9]

Correct answer is A – Cerebellar infarction

This patient has signs consistent with a left cerebellar infarct. Cerebellar strokes produce ipsilateral signs. This is confirmed by the changes found in the CT scan. Ischaemic changes are normally reported as areas of 'low attenuation' compared with haemorrhages, which are seen as dense white areas.[1,9]

Some of the signs of cerebellar infarction can be remembered using the mnemonic 'DANISH':

• **D**ysdiadochokinesis
• **A**taxia
• **N**ystagmus
• **I**ntention tremor

- **S**canning dysarthria
- **H**ypotonia/positive **H**eel shin test.

A10

Correct answer is B – Infarct of the left internal capsule

The patient has most likely suffered a lacunar infarct. He has a pure motor right-sided hemiparesis. Lacunar infarcts are caused by occlusion of the lenticulostriate arteries (derived from the middle cerebral artery) that supply the basal ganglia and internal capsule. There is a variety of syndromes associated with lacunar infarction including pure motor, pure sensory, mixed sensorimotor, ataxic hemiparesis and dysarthria-clumsy hand syndrome.

This patient most likely suffered an infarction of the posterior limb of the left internal capsule. If he had an infarction of the lateral thalamus, then he would have most likely presented with pure sensory symptoms. If he had infarction of the thalamus and internal capsule (thalamocapsular infarction) then it is likely his symptoms would be sensorimotor.[1,9] His glucose and blood pressure are well controlled, meaning that trauma from a hypoglycaemic fall (answer E) can be excluded.

References

1. Kumar PJ, Clark ML, editors. *Kumar & Clark's Clinical Medicine.* 7th ed. Edinburgh: Saunders Elsevier; 2009.
2. Akhtar N, Kamran SI, Deleu D, *et al.* Ischaemic posterior circulation stroke in State of Qatar. *Eur J Neurol.* 2009; **16**(9): 1004–9.
3. Crossman AR, Neary D. *Neuroanatomy: an illustrated colour text.* 3rd ed. Edinburgh: Elsevier; 2005.
4. Finelli PF. Neuroimaging in acute posterior cerebral artery infarction. *Neurologist.* 2008; **14**(3): 170–80.
5. Kobayashi S, Maki T, Kunimoto M. Clinical symptoms of bilateral anterior cerebral artery territory infarction. *J Clin Neurosci.* 2011; **18**(2): 218–22.
6. Droste DW, Ritter MA, Dittrich R, *et al.* Arterial hypertension and ischaemic stroke. *Acta Neurol Scand.* 2003; **107**(4): 241–51.
7. Fauci A, Braunwald E, Kasper D, *et al.*, editors. *Harrison's Principles of Internal Medicine.* 17th ed. New York, NY: McGraw-Hill; 2008.
8. Longmore M, Wilkinson IB, Davidson EH, *et al. Oxford Handbook of Clinical Medicine.* 8th ed. New York, NY: Oxford University Press; 2010.

9. Fitzgerald MJT, Gruener G, Mtui E. *Clinical Neuroanatomy and Neuroscience*. 5th ed. Edinburgh: Elsevier Saunders; 2007.

10. Chou CL, Lin YJ, Sheu YL, *et al*. Persistent Klüver–Bucy syndrome after bilateral temporal lobe infarction. *Acta Neurol Taiwan*. 2008; **17**(3): 199–202.

11. National Institute for Health and Care Excellence. Stroke: diagnosis and initial management of acute stroke and transient ischaemic attack (TIA); NICE guideline 68. London: NICE; 2008. http://publications.nice.org.uk/stroke-cg68

12. Goljan EF. *Rapid Review Pathology*. 3rd ed. Philadelphia, PA: Mosby/Elsevier; 2010.

Index

CPD with Radcliffe

You can now use a selection of our books to achieve CPD (Continuing Professional Development) points through directed reading.

We provide a free online form and downloadable certificate for your appraisal portfolio. Look for the CPD logo and register with us at: www.radcliffehealth.com/cpd

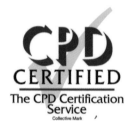